THE DASH DIET
FOOD LIST

BY MORGAN F. WHITTAKER

LEGAL & DISCLAIMER

The information contained in this book is not designed to replace or take the place of any form of medicine or professional medical advice. The information in this book has been provided for educational and entertainment purposes only.

You need to consult a professional medical practitioner in order to ensure you are both healthy enough and able to make use of this information. Always consult your professional medical practitioner before undertaking any new dietary regime, and particularly after reading this book.

The information contained in this book has been compiled from sources deemed reliable, and it is accurate to the best of the Author's knowledge; however, the Author cannot guarantee its accuracy and validity and cannot be held liable for any errors or omissions.

You must consult your doctor or get professional medical advice before using any suggested information in this book.

Upon using the information contained in this book, you agree to hold harmless the Author, and Publisher, from and against any damages, costs, and expenses, including any legal fees potentially resulting from the application of any of the information provided by this guide. This disclaimer applies to any damages or injury caused by the use and application, whether directly or indirectly, of any advice or information presented, whether for breach of contract, tort, negligence, personal injury, criminal intent, or under any other cause of action. You agree to accept all risks of using the information presented inside this book.

CONTENTS

INTRODUCTION..7

WHAT EVEN IS THE DASH DIET? 9

HOW TO USE THIS FOOD LIST 13

SOURCES 15

THE FOOD LIST 17

INTRODUCTION

Congratulations on choosing this book.

Let's start with the basics. DASH (Dietary Approaches to Stop Hypertension) is a flexible and balanced eating plan. You don't need anything fancy for it, just good, healthy ingredients that can help you get healthy.

The WHO estimates 1.28 billion adults aged 30-79 years have hypertension and approximately 21% with hypertension have it under control.

Hypertension is caused by unhealthy lifestyle choices such as too much salt in the diet, a lack of exercise, smoking, too much alcohol, stress, old age and genes (source: *Web MD*).

According to the CDC, it is possible to lower blood pressure into a healthy range by making lifestyle changes such as eating a low-sodium diet.

I wrote this book because I want to help those with hypertension eat a healthier diet and lower blood pressure and I was frustrated at how so much information out there seems to completely contradict other sources.

Essentially, some of the top DASH resources aren't very clear. There's a lot of spammy, low-quality books out there that disagree with each other. Which is not very helpful. One will tell you something is allowed on the DASH diet, and another will tell you it is not.

I believe diet plays a huge part in living a healthy lifestyle and it is possible to prevent and control hypertension by making better food choices.

So I decided to research the web and combine the most trusted DASH guides and compile the information into one easy-to-consult food list, *that you can take everywhere*.

Trust me, it's been quite the process.

WHAT EVEN IS THE DASH DIET?

The DASH diet was first introduced in 1997. Since then, it has been promoted by the National Institute of Health's National Heart, Lung, and Blood Institute for reducing blood pressure.

DASH is a balanced plan that may also help with aid weight loss, lower risk of diabetes, heart disease and cancer.

The standard DASH diet limits sodium to **2,300 mg (approx. six grams of salt**) a day. The lower sodium version of the DASH diet limits sodium even further to **1,500 mg (approx. four grams of salt**) a day (*source: Mayo Clinic*). If you're unsure of which plan to follow, speak to your doctor.

When following the DASH eating plan, the US department of Health and Human Services tells to eat foods that are:

- *Low in saturated and* trans fats
- *Rich in potassium, calcium, magnesium, fiber, and protein*
- *Lower in sodium (source: US Dept of Health and Human Services)*

And avoiding fatty meats, full-fat dairy sweet drinks, sweets and sodium intake (*source: NHLBI*).

Heart & Stroke's website lists the DASH diet food groups as the following with recommended servings next to each:

- Vegetables (4-5 servings)
- Fruit (4-5 servings)
- Grains (mainly whole grains) (7-8 servings)
- Low fat or no-fat dairy foods (2-3 servings)
- Lean meats, poultry and fish (2 servings or less)
- Nuts, seeds and dry beans (4-5 servings per week)
- Fats and oils (2-3 servings)

Note the serving amounts will depend on age, gender and activity levels.

Heart & Stroke's website also noted:

"At every meal fill half your plate with vegetables and fruit, a quarter of your plate with whole-grain foods, and a quarter of your plate with protein foods."

The importance of limiting sodium intake was demonstrated in a study by the DASH-Sodium Collaborative Research Group.

A study was done on 412 participants who were randomly assigned to eat a typical US diet or the DASH diet. The participants ate foods with high, intermediate and low levels of sodium for 30 days.

They found:

"Reducing the sodium intake from the high to the intermediate level reduced the systolic blood pressure by 2.1 mm Hg (P<0.001) during the control diet and by 1.3 mm Hg (P=0.03) during the DASH diet. Reducing the sodium intake from the intermediate to the low level caused additional reductions of 4.6 mm Hg during the control diet (P<0.001) and 1.7 mm Hg during the DASH diet (P<0.01)."

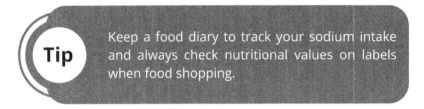

Tip Keep a food diary to track your sodium intake and always check nutritional values on labels when food shopping.

Whilst the DASH diet does help lower blood pressure, the study also concluded *"long-term health benefits will depend on the ability of people to make long-lasting dietary changes and the increased availability of lower-sodium foods."*

I believe this list is the most comprehensive out there, and where there is debate, I have deferred to many of the top sources listed in these pages. With all that said, there will be areas you disagree on and that is why a) approach any new food with caution, and b) always consult your medical practitioner before making any dietary changes.

I know this list will never be definitive, nutritional values may vary from brand to brand and I will continue to refine it as more information becomes available.

This isn't the place to speculate on why you are on the DASH diet in the first place. I'm sure you've done your research. No, you're here because you want the best DASH diet food information book, at your fingertips.

Use this book to avoid foods that are high in saturated fats, sugar-sweetened in some way or high in sodium. These can include foods you wouldn't expect to find - more on that later.

It's also important to point out that not everybody needs to follow dietary approaches to stop hypertension, nor wants to. All of which means you should consult with your practitioner to determine the correct course for you. Please keep in mind that materials and resources like this book are no substitute for medical advice and not intended as such.

Now, let's get straight onto the list.

HOW TO USE THIS FOOD LIST

This book works like a dictionary. Look for a food, drink or ingredient alphabetically or on search.

Once you find what you are looking for, you'll find the following nutritional values **per 100 grams** based on the USDA database (unless stated otherwise);

Saturated fat content
Sodium content

Sugar content

And then assorted notes.

So I've made it more straightforward in this book. I've consulted those sites, and each food then gets a symbol.

✓ = consume more of this on the DASH diet

☺ = Limit on the DASH diet

So on the DASH diet, you would look to consume more ✔ foods and less ☠ foods. It's simple really.

The DASH diet isn't a quick-fix solution. The purpose of this diet is to promote heart health, eat better and incorporate this diet into your life in the long run so you live a happy and healthy life.

It should be pointed out that respected sites sometimes disagree on major foods so I've tried to reflect that in this list.

At this point, a disclaimer. The aim is to meticulously study the research, learn more about the DASH diet, and live a healthy, balanced life in every aspect. This book has been a labour of love, but it has been a challenge to put together as the major lists sometimes disagree on how to approach the DASH diet.

Consult your doctor or get professional medical advice before using the information in this book. This is a guide, not a definitive list as everybody is individual.

So work with an expert, and this book close by when you cook or eat out, and dip in and out whenever you need to check if something is DASH compliant!

SOURCES

These excellent sources come highly recommended in your further research on the DASH diet. Please do click on these resources and sites for further reading. I consider them to be the best sources out there.

- Mayo Clinic - DASH diet: healthy eating to lower your blood pressure https://www.mayoclinic.org/healthy-life-style/nutrition-and-healthy-eating/in-depth/dash-diet/art-20048456#:~:text=The%20DASH%20diet%20is%20rich,and%20full%2Dfat%20dairy%20products.

- National Heart, Lung and Blood Institute (NIH) - DASH eating plan: https://www.nhlbi.nih.gov/education/dash-eating-plan

- Pub Med - Effects of blood pressure of reduced dietary sodium and the Dietary Approaches to Stop Hypertension (DASH) diet. DASH-Sodium Collaborative Research Group https://pubmed.ncbi.nlm.nih.gov/11136953/

- Trifecta Nutrition - DASH Diet Guidelines and Food Lists https://www.trifectanutrition.com/health/dash-diet-guidelines-and-food-lists

- National Heart, Lung and Blood Institute (NIH) - Your guide to lowering your blood pressure with DASH - https://www.nhlbi.nih.gov/files/docs/public/heart/new_dash.pdf

- FDA - Sodium in your diet - https://www.fda.gov/food/nutrition-education-resources-materials/sodium-your-diet

- NHS - Sugar: the facts - https://www.nhs.uk/live-well/eat-well/how-does-sugar-in-our-diet-affect-our-health/

- Cleveland Clinic - Sodium controlled diet - https://my.clevelandclinic.org/health/articles/15426-sodium-controlled-diet

THE FOOD LIST

Aim for:

➢ Foods **less than five percent** of the daily value of sodium
➢ **Less than 140mg** of sodium per serving
➢ **One gram or less** per serving of saturated fat
➢ **Less than five grams** of sugar per 100g

(sources: *NIH, FDA, NHS*)

Acerola:

➢ Saturated fat content: 0.1g (per 100g) ✔
➢ Sodium content: 7mg (per 100g), less than 1% daily value based on a 2,000 calorie diet ✔
➢ Sugar content: Not reported by the USDA however, a 1-cup serving of raw acerola juice contains 11g of sugar (source: *Livestrong*). ☹

Also known as *Barbados Cherries*. Acerola is low in saturated fat and sodium content however, acerola juice is high in sugar so avoid juicing this fruit.

Agave syrup:

➢ Saturated fat content: 0g (per 100g) ✔
➢ Sodium content: 4mg (per 100g), less than 1% daily value based on a 2,000 calorie diet ✔
➢ Sugar content: 68g (per 100g) ☠

Also known as *agave nectar*. Low in sodium and saturated fat but thought to be high in sugar content. Avoid on the DASH diet.

Alcohol:

➢ Saturated fat content: 0g (per 100g) ✔
➢ Sodium content: 4mg (per 100g), less than 1% daily value based on a 2,000 calorie diet ✔
➢ Sugar content: 0g (per 100g) ✔

Alcohol generally is low in saturated fat, sodium and sugar content. The sugar content will vary depending on the type of alcohol so I recommend you check the nutritional values for each drink carefully.

Healthline recommends drinking alcohol sparingly on the DASH diet. You don't have to eliminate alcohol completely although it's good to limit consumption.

PubMed have published a study concluding:

"A high DASH score and a reduction in alcohol consumption could be effective nutritional strategies for the prevention of hypertension."

Another study by the U.S. Department of Veteran Affairs found:

"Participants who increased their alcohol intake also increased their rate of unhealthy eating."

Algae:

- ➤ Saturated fat content: 2g (per 100g) 💀
- ➤ Sodium content: 812mg (per 100g), 35% daily value based on a 2,000 calorie diet 💀
- ➤ Sugar content: 3.07g (per 100g) ✔

Low in sugar but thought to be high in saturated fat and sodium content. Avoid on the DASH diet.

Almond:

- ➤ Saturated fat content: 3.8g (per 100g) 💀
- ➤ Sodium content: 1mg (per 100g), less than 1% daily value based on a 2,000 calorie diet ✔
- ➤ Sugar content: 4.35g (per 100g) ✔

Almonds may be enjoyed as part of a healthy diet. Eating Well's website notes almonds as part of the DASH diet and a heart-healthy lifestyle. Ensure you eat no more than 4-5 servings a week.

PubMed have published a study concluding:

"Almonds might have a considerable favorite effect in blood pressure and especially in diastolic blood pressure, and it could be encouraged

as part of a healthy diet; however due to the high calorie content, the intake should be part of healthy diet."

Anchovies:

➤ Saturated fat content: 2.2g (per 100g) ☻
➤ Sodium content: 3,668 mg (per 100g), 152% daily value based on a 2,000 calorie diet ☻
➤ Sugar content: 0g (per 100g) ✔

Low in sugar but thought to be high in saturated fat and sodium content. Avoid on the DASH diet.

Apple:

➤ Saturated fat content: 0g (per 100g) ✔
➤ Sodium content: 1mg (per 100g), less than 1% daily value based on a 2,000 calorie diet ✔
➤ Sugar content: 10g (per 100g) ☻

Note the high sugar content. Eat in moderation.

Apple cider vinegar:

➤ Saturated fat content: 0g (per 100g) ✔
➤ Sodium content: 5mg (per 100g), less than 1% daily value based on a 2,000 calorie diet ✔
➤ Sugar content: 0.4g (per 100g) ✔

Allowed on the DASH diet. Studies have shown apple cider vinegar to lower post-meal blood glucose (source: *The University of Chicago Medical Center*).

Apricot:

➢ Saturated fat content: 0g (per 100g) ✔
➢ Sodium content: 1mg (per 100g), less than 1% daily value based on a 2,000 calorie diet ✔
➢ Sugar content: 9g (per 100g) 😕

Low in saturated fat and sodium content but high in sugar. Eat in moderation.

Artichokes:

➢ Saturated fat content: 0g (per 100g) ✔
➢ Sodium content: 94mg (per 100g), 3% daily value based on a 2,000 calorie diet ✔
➢ Sugar content: 1g (per 100g) ✔

Allowed on the DASH diet. A study found artichoke leaf juice contained antihypertensive effect in patients with mild hypertension (source: *PubMed*).

Artificial sweeteners:

➢ Saturated fat content: 0g (per 100g) ✔
➢ Sodium content: 572mg (per 100g), 23% daily value based on a 2,000 calorie diet 😕
➢ Sugar content: 4g (per 100g) ✔

It's thought that using sugar alternatives such as stevia and Splenda are acceptable on this diet however, you might avoid artificial sweeteners due to the potential negative effects on your gut microbiome. If you can, using natural sweeteners such as Stevia is preferable.

Asparagus:

➤ Saturated fat content: 0g (per 100g) ✔
➤ Sodium content: 2mg (per 100g), less than 1% daily value based on a 2,000 calorie diet ✔
➤ Sugar content: 1.9g (per 100g) ✔

Allowed on the DASH diet. Consume 4-5 servings of vegetables a day.

Aubergine:

➤ Saturated fat content: 0g (per 100g) ✔
➤ Sodium content: 2mg (per 100g), less than 1% daily value based on a 2,000 calorie diet ✔
➤ Sugar content: 3.5g (per 100g) ✔

Allowed on the DASH diet. Aubergines are also a great source of fiber. A study found aubergines can control diabetes through their anti-oxidative properties.

Consume 4-5 servings of vegetables a day. (That's a mantra you'll hear time and again on the DASH diet).

(source: *Yarmohammadi F, Ghasemzadeh Rahbardar M, Hosseinzadeh H. Effect of eggplant (Solanum melongena) on the metabolic syndrome*)

Avocado:

➢ Saturated fat content: 2.1g (per 100g) ☻
➢ Sodium content: 7mg (per 100g), less than 1% daily value based on a 2,000 calorie diet ✓
➢ Sugar content: 0.7g (per 100g) ✓

Allowed on the DASH diet. Avocados are a great source of potassium which is great for your heart. They may also lower your blood pressure (source: *Hello Heart*).

Whilst avocado is healthy, it's still higher in fat compared to other fruits.

Bamboo shoots:

➢ Saturated fat content: 0.1g (per 100g) ✓
➢ Sodium content: 4mg (per 100g), less than 1% daily value based on a 2,000 calorie diet ✓
➢ Sugar content: 3g (per 100g) ✓

Allowed on the DASH diet. Note that bamboo shoots should never be consumed raw or unprocessed due to natural toxins present which may cause health problems.

(Source: *Nongdam P, Tikendra L. The Nutritional Facts of Bamboo Shoots and Their Usage as Important Traditional Foods of Northeast India*).

Banana:

➢ Saturated fat content: 0.1g (per 100g) ✔
➢ Sodium content: 1mg (per 100g) ✔
➢ Sugar content: 12g (per 100g) 💀

Low in saturated fat and sodium content but high in sugar. Eat in moderation.

Barley:

➢ Saturated fat content: 0.5g (per 100g) ✔
➢ Sodium content: 12mg (per 100g), less than 1% daily value based on a 2,000 calorie diet ✔
➢ Sugar content: 0.8g (per 100g) ✔

Allowed on the DASH diet. Evidence shows barley reduces blood pressure (source: *Oldways Whole Grains Council*).

Basil:

➢ Saturated fat content: 0g (per 100g) ✔
➢ Sodium content: 4mg (per 100g), less than 1% daily value based on a 2,000 calorie diet ✔
➢ Sugar content: 0.3g (per 100g) ✔

Allowed on the DASH diet. PubMed have published a study on the role of herbs in treating hypertension. They found basil causes a fall in systolic, diastolic, and mean blood pressure.

(source: *Tabassum N, Ahmad F. Role of natural herbs in the treatment of hypertension. Pharmacogn Rev*)

Beans:

➢ Saturated fat content: 0.2g (per 100g) ✔
➢ Sodium content: 12mg (per 100g), less than 1% daily value based on a 2,000 calorie diet ✔
➢ Sugar content: 2.1g (per 100g) ✔

Allowed on the DASH diet. Ensure you eat no more than 4-5 servings a week.

Beef:

➢ Saturated fat content: 6g (per 100g) ☠
➢ Sodium content: 72mg (per 100g), 3% daily value based on a 2,000 calorie diet ✔
➢ Sugar content: 0g (per 100g) ✔

Must be grass-fed beef as grain-fed beef contributes to inflammation and heart disease (source: *Medicine Net*). Eat no more than 2 servings a day.

Beer:

➢ Saturated fat content: 0g (per 100g) ✔
➢ Sodium content: 4mg, less than 1% daily value based on a 2,000 calorie diet ✔
➢ Sugar content: 0g (per 100g) ✔

Drink alcohol sparingly on the DASH diet. You don't have to eliminate alcohol completely although it's good to limit consumption.

Beetroot:

➢ Saturated fat content: 0g (per 100g) ✔
➢ Sodium content: 78mg (per 100g), 3% daily value based on a 2,000 calorie diet ✔
➢ Sugar content: 7g (per 100g) ☹

Also known as *Beets*. This lovely veg contains nitrates — natural chemicals which help promote blood flow. Studies have shown nitrates "*acutely lowers blood pressure*". Consume 4-5 servings of vegetables a day.

(Source: *Hobbs DA, George TW, Lovegrove JA. The effects of dietary nitrate on blood pressure and endothelial function: a review of human intervention studies*)

Bell pepper (hot):

➢ Saturated fat content: 0g (per 100g) ✔
➢ Sodium content: 9mg (per 100g), less than 1% daily value based on a 2,000 calorie diet ✔
➢ Sugar content: 5g (per 100g) ✔

Allowed on the DASH diet. They're also a great source of vitamin C. Half a cup of raw red pepper is thought to contain 95mg of vitamin C, which is 106% of the daily value (source: *Medical News*

Today). Consume 4-5 servings of vegetables a day and don't forget to add this to your diet plan.

Bell pepper (sweet):

➢ Saturated fat content: 0g (per 100g) ✔
➢ Sodium content: 4mg (per 100g), less than 1% daily value based on a 2,000 calorie diet ✔
➢ Sugar content: 4.2g (per 100g) ✔

Allowed on the DASH diet. They're also a great source of vitamin C. Half a cup of raw red pepper is thought to contain 95mg of vitamin C, which is 106% of the daily value (source: *Medical News Today*). Consume 4-5 servings of vegetables a day and don't forget to add this to your diet plan.

Bison:

➢ Saturated fat content: 0.69g (per 100g) ✔
➢ Sodium content: 54mg (per 100g), 2% daily value based on a 2,000 calorie diet ✔
➢ Sugar content: 0g (per 100g) ✔

Allowed on the DASH diet. The American Heart Association also recommends bison. Consume no more than 2 servings a day.

Bivalves (mussels, oyster, clams, scallops):

Let's dig into these different seafoods and discuss whether they are suitable on the DASH diet.

Mussels:

➢ Saturated fat content: 0.9g (per 100g) ✔
➢ Sodium content: 369mg (per 100g), 15% daily value based on a 2,000 calorie diet ☹
➢ Sugar content: 0g (per 100g) ✔

High in sodium. Avoid.

Oysters:

➢ Saturated fat content: 3.2g (per 100g) ☹
➢ Sodium content: 417mg (per 100g), 17% daily value based on a 2,000 calorie diet ☹
➢ Sugar content: 0g (per 100g) ✔

Low in sugar but thought to be high in saturated fat and sodium content. Avoid.

Clams (source: *nutritionix*):

➢ Saturated fat content: 0.2g (per 100g) ✔
➢ Sodium content: 1,202mg (per 100g), 50% daily value based on a 2,000 calorie diet ☹
➢ Sugar content: 0g (per 100g) ✔

High in sodium. Avoid.

Scallops:

➢ Saturated fat content: 0.2g (per 100g) ✔

- ➢ Sodium content: 667mg (per 100g), 27% daily value based on a 2,000 calorie diet ☠
- ➢ Sugar content: 0g (per 100g) ✓

High in sodium. Avoid.

Black caraway:

- ➢ Saturated fat content: 0.5g (per 100g) ✓
- ➢ Sodium content: 88mg (per 100g), 3% daily value based on a 2,000 calorie diet ✓
- ➢ Sugar content: 0.64g (per 100g) ✓

Allowed on the DASH diet.

Blackberry:

- ➢ Saturated fat content: 0g (per 100g) ✓
- ➢ Sodium content: 1mg (per 100g), less than 1% daily value based on a 2,000 calorie diet ✓
- ➢ Sugar content: 4.9g (per 100g) ✓

Allowed on the DASH diet. This superfood is supposedly great for the brain and it helps to reduce blood pressure (source: *Urology of Virginia*).

Blackcurrants:

- ➢ Saturated fat content: 0.034g (per 100g) ✓
- ➢ Sodium content: 2mg (per 100g), less than 1% daily value based on a 2,000 calorie diet ✓
- ➢ Sugar content: 0g (per 100g) ✓

Allowed on the DASH diet. Try not to eat too much if you're also taking medication to lower blood pressure because blackcurrants may lower your blood pressure further (source: *webMD*).

Blue cheeses:

➢ Saturated fat content: 19g (per 100g) 😨
➢ Sodium content: 1,395mg (per 100g), 58% daily value based on a 2,000 calorie diet 😨
➢ Sugar content: 0.5g (per 100g) ✔

Low in sugar but generally high in saturated fat and sodium content. Avoid on the DASH diet.

Blueberries:

➢ Saturated fat content: 0g (per 100g) ✔
➢ Sodium content: 1mg (per 100g), less than 1% daily value based on a 2,000 calorie diet ✔
➢ Sugar content: 10g (per 100g) ✔

Allowed on the DASH diet. Harvard's website notes:

"Consuming 200 grams of blueberries (about one cup) daily can improve blood vessel function and decrease systolic blood pressure."

Bok choi:

➢ Saturated fat content: 0g (per 100g) ✔
➢ Sodium content: 65mg (per 100g), 2% daily value based on a 2,000 calorie diet ✔
➢ Sugar content: 1.2g ✔

Sometimes also written as *bok choy* or *Chinese cabbage*. A lovely leafy green veg. Try sautéing or lightly roasting for 15 minutes. Researchers found sulforaphane (the active ingredient in bok choi) helps to reduce blood pressure (source: *OHSU Research News*). Allowed on the DASH diet.

Borlotti beans:

- ➢ Saturated fat content: 0.3g (per 100g) ✔
- ➢ Sodium content: 0mg (per 100g) ✔
- ➢ Sugar content: 0.83g (per 100g) ✔

Also known as the *cranberry bean*. Allowed on the DASH diet but ensure you eat no more than 4-5 servings a week.

Bouillon:

- ➢ Saturated fat content: 3.4g (per 100g) ☺
- ➢ Sodium content: 23,875mg (per 100g), 994% daily value based on a 2,000 calorie diet ☺
- ➢ Sugar content: 17g (per 100g) ☺

Also known as *broth*. Broth is made from simmering water with either meat, fish or seafood. It tends to be high in sodium so avoid.

Boysenberry:

- ➢ Saturated fat content: 0.014g (per 100g) ✔
- ➢ Sodium content: 0mg (per 100g) ✔
- ➢ Sugar content: 4.88g (per 100g) ✔

A cross of loganberry, blackberry and raspberry. Boysenberry is another super fruit that is full of potassium and magnesium. It has been found to reduce blood pressure. Allowed on the DASH diet.

Brandy:

➢ Saturated fat content: 0g (per 100g) ✔
➢ Sodium content: 1mg (per 100g), less than 1% daily value based on a 2,000 calorie diet ✔
➢ Sugar content: 0g (per 100g) ✔

Whilst brandy is allowed on the DASH diet, as with all alcohol, drink in moderation as too much alcohol will raise blood pressure.

Brazil nut:

➢ Saturated fat content: 15g (per 100g) ☻
➢ Sodium content: 3mg (per 100g), less than 1% daily value based on a 2,000 calorie diet ✔
➢ Sugar content: 2.3g (per 100g) ✔

They're also high in potassium. Ensure you eat no more than 4-5 servings a week and go for unsalted nuts. Serving size can be a challenge with nuts.

Bread:

➢ Saturated fat content: 0.7g (per 100g) ✔
➢ Sodium content: 491mg, 20% daily value based on a 2,000 calorie diet (per 100g) ☻
➢ Sugar content: 5g (per 100g) ✔

High in sodium. Unfortunately, this staple food is the top contributor of dietary sodium in the US (source: *Vox*). Limit intake.

Broad-leaved garlic:

➢ Saturated fat content: 0.089g (per 100g) ✔
➢ Sodium content: 17mg (per 100g), 1% daily value based on a 2,000 calorie diet ✔
➢ Sugar content: 1g (per 100g) ✔

This guide has used the nutritional values for garlic as the USDA and other sources do not list the nutritional values for broad-leaved garlic. Allowed on the DASH diet.

Broad beans:

➢ Saturated fat content: 0.1g (per 100g) ✔
➢ Sodium content: 25mg (per 100g), 1% daily value based on a 2,000 calorie diet ✔
➢ Sugar content: 9g (per 100g) 💀

Also known as *Vicia Faba*. Low in saturated fat and sodium content but high in sugar. Eat in moderation. Ensure you eat no more than 4-5 servings a week.

Broccoli:

➢ Saturated fat content: 0.039g (per 100g) ✔
➢ Sodium content: 33mg (per 100g), less than 1% daily value based on a 2,000 calorie diet ✔
➢ Sugar content: 1.7g (per 100g) ✔

Allowed on the DASH diet. It's rich in vitamin C, folate and fiber. Researchers found sulforaphane (the active ingredient in broccoli) helps to reduce blood pressure (source: *OHSU Research News*). Consume 4-5 servings of vegetables a day.

Brussels sprouts:

➢ Saturated fat content: 0.1g (per 100g) ✔
➢ Sodium content: 25mg (per 100g), 1% daily value based on a 2,000 calorie diet ✔
➢ Sugar content: 2.2g (per 100g) ✔

Allowed on the DASH diet. One cup of Brussels sprouts contains roughly 350mg of potassium (source: *Unity Point*). Eat 4-5 servings of vegetables a day.

Buckwheat:

➢ Saturated fat content: 0.741g (per 100g) ✔
➢ Sodium content: 1mg (per 100g), less than 1% daily value based on a 2,000 calorie diet ✔
➢ Sugar content: N/A (per 100g) ✔

Allowed on the DASH diet. It's gluten free and according to Olga In The Kitchen's blog, it's just as simple to prepare as white rice.

Butter:

➢ Saturated fat content: 51g (per 100g) ☹
➢ Sodium content: 11mg (per 100g), less than 1% daily value based on a 2,000 calorie diet ✔
➢ Sugar content: 0.1g (per 100g) ✔

WebMD suggests using low-fat or fat-free butter and halving your usual serving. Mayo Clinic notes *"margarine usually tops butter when it comes to heart health"*. As butter comes from animal fat, there's more saturated fat. If you want to have butter, make sure it is unsalted too.

Cabbage:

➢ Saturated fat content: 0g (per 100g) ✔
➢ Sodium content: 18mg (per 100g), less than 1% daily value based on a 2,000 calorie diet ✔
➢ Sugar content: 3.2g (per 100g) ✔

Allowed on the DASH diet. Cabbage is thought to contain high levels of potassium which may help lower blood pressure. Consume 4-5 servings of vegetables a day.

Cactus pear:

➢ Saturated fat content: 0.1g (per 100g) ✔
➢ Sodium content: 5mg (per 100g), less than 1% daily value based on a 2,000 calorie diet ✔
➢ Sugar content: N/A (per 100g) ✔

Allowed on the DASH diet. Consume 4-5 servings of vegetables a day. According to Mayo Clinic, cactus pears are promoted for treating diabetes, high cholesterol, obesity and hangovers. Enjoy as part of a healthy diet.

Cardamom:

➢ Saturated fat content: 0.7g (per 100g) ✔

➢ Sodium content: 18mg (per 100g), less than 1% daily value based on a 2,000 calorie diet ✔
➢ Sugar content: N/A (per 100g) ✔

Seeds from the cardamon plant. A number of sources outline the benefits of cardamom and even call it *"the Queen Spices"*. A study found *"antibacterial and anti-inflammatory properties"* of cardamom against periodontal infections.

Allowed on the DASH diet.

(source: *Souissi M, Azelmat J, Chaieb K, Grenier D. Antibacterial and anti-inflammatory activities of cardamom (Elettaria cardamomum) extracts: Potential therapeutic benefits for periodontal infections*)

Carrot:

➢ Saturated fat content: 0g (per 100g) ✔
➢ Sodium content: 69mg (per 100g), 2% daily value based on a 2,000 calorie diet ✔
➢ Sugar content: 4.7g (per 100g) ✔

Allowed on the DASH diet. It's thought that eating carrots raw may be more beneficial in reducing blood pressure (source: *Health-line*). Consume 4-5 servings of vegetables a day.

Cashew nut:

➢ Saturated fat content: 8g (per 100g) 😷

- ➢ Sodium content: 12mg (per 100g), less than 1% daily value based on a 2,000 calorie diet ✔
- ➢ Sugar content: 6g (per 100g) 😵

Cashew nuts are high in saturated fat and whilst the DASH diet recommends eating foods that are low in saturated fat, almonds are a source of good saturated fat which is thought to be linked to better cholesterol levels (source: *Insider*).

Eat no more than 4-5 servings a week and go for unsalted nuts.

Cassava:

- ➢ Saturated fat content: 0.1g (per 100g) ✔
- ➢ Sodium content: 14mg (per 100g), less than 1% daily value based on a 2,000 calorie diet ✔
- ➢ Sugar content: 1.7g (per 100g) ✔

Allowed on the DASH diet. High in potassium as a cup of cassava is thought to contain 558mg which is 16% to 21% of the daily recommendation (source: *verywellfit*). Why not have cassava on the side instead of grains?

Cauliflower:

- ➢ Saturated fat content: 0.1g (per 100g) ✔
- ➢ Sodium content: 30mg (per 100g), 1% daily value based on a 2,000 calorie diet ✔
- ➢ Sugar content: 1.9g (per 100g) ✔

Allowed on the DASH diet. Researchers found sulforaphane (the active ingredient in cauliflower) helps to reduce blood pressure (source: *OHSU Research News*). Eat 4-5 servings of vegetables a day.

Celery:

➢ Saturated fat content: 0.042g (per 100g) ✔
➢ Sodium content: 80mg (per 100g), 3% daily value based on a 2,000 calorie diet ✔
➢ Sugar content: 1.34 g (per 100g) ✔

Celery sticks are great as a quick healthy snack. Just make sure to check the nutritional values of any sauce you use.

Allowed on the DASH diet and eat 4-5 servings of vegetables a day.

Cep mushrooms:

➢ Saturated fat content: 3.1g (per 100g) ☹
➢ Sodium content: 304mg (per 100g), 12% daily value based on a 2,000 calorie diet ☹
➢ Sugar content: 32g (per 100g) ☹

Also known as *Penny Bun*. The values based on the USDA's database suggests this mushroom is high in saturated fat, sodium and sugar content. Avoid.

Chamomile and chamomile tea:

➢ Saturated fat content: 0.002g (per 100g) ✔

- ➢ Sodium content: 1mg (per 100g), less than 1% daily value based on a 2,000 calorie diet ✔
- ➢ Sugar content: 0g (per 100g) ✔

Allowed on the DASH diet. It's thought that chamomile may lower blood pressure.

Champagne:

- ➢ Saturated fat content: 0g (per 100g) ✔
- ➢ Sodium content: 5mg (per 100g), less than 1% daily value based on a 2,000 calorie diet ✔
- ➢ Sugar content: 0.79g (per 100g) ✔

Allowed on the DASH diet. Drink alcohol sparingly on the DASH diet. You don't have to eliminate champagne completely although it's good to limit consumption.

The University of Reading found champagne may be good for your heart and circulation by increasing the availability of nitric oxide therefore, improving the functioning of your blood vessels.

Chard:

- ➢ Saturated fat content: 0.03g (per 100g) ✔
- ➢ Sodium content: 213mg (per 100g), 9% daily value based on a 2,000 calorie diet ☹
- ➢ Sugar content: 1.1g (per 100g) ✔

Chard is naturally higher in sodium than other vegetables. It's thought to contain high levels of nitrates which helps reduce blood pressure (source: *Medical News Today*).

Cheddar cheese:

➢ Saturated fat content: 21g (per 100g) ☠
➢ Sodium content: 621mg (per 100g), 25% daily value based on a 2,000 calorie diet ☠
➢ Sugar content: 0.5g (per 100g) ✔

Low in sugar but thought to be high in saturated fat and sodium content. Cheddar is a processed and hard cheese. Avoid on the DASH diet.

Cheese made from unpasteurized "raw" milk:

➢ Saturated fat content: 14.3g (per 100g) ☠
➢ Sodium content: 482mg (per 100g), 21% daily value based on a 2,000 calorie diet ☠
➢ Sugar content: 0g (per 100g) ✔

(source: *Eat this much*)

I've based the above on raw milk cheddar cheese. Low in sugar but thought to be high in saturated fat and sodium content.

Cheeses:

➢ Saturated fat content: 21g (per 100g) ☠

➢ Sodium content: 621mg (per 100g), 25% daily value based on a 2,000 calorie diet 💀
➢ Sugar content: 0.5g (per 100g) ✔

Cheese in general is thought to be low in sugar but high in saturated fat and sodium content.

Check the nutritional labels for each cheese. Cleveland Clinic recommends going for naturally low-sodium cheese such as Swiss, goat, brick ricotta and fresh mozzarella. Avoid processed and hard cheeses.

Cherry:

➢ Saturated fat content: 0.1g (per 100g) ✔
➢ Sodium content: 3mg (per 100g), less than 1% daily value based on a 2,000 calorie diet ✔
➢ Sugar content: 8g (per 100g) 💀

Low in saturated fat and sodium content but high in sugar. Interestingly, a study found drinking tart cherry juice lowers LDL cholesterol and total cholesterol. The study noted longer follow-up studies are needed to further assess the benefits.

(source: *Chai SC , Davis K , Wright RS , Kuczmarski MF , Zhang Z . Impact of tart cherry juice on systolic blood pressure and low-density lipoprotein cholesterol in older adults: a randomized controlled trial*)

Chia, chia seeds:

➢ Saturated fat content: 3.3g (per 100g) ☠
➢ Sodium content: 16mg (per 100g), less than 1% daily value based on a 2,000 calorie diet ✔
➢ Sugar content: N/A (per 100g) ✔

Eat no more than 4-5 servings a week. Eating Well's website notes chia seeds as part of the DASH diet and a heart-healthy lifestyle.

Chicken:

➢ Saturated fat content: 3.8g (per 100g) ☠
➢ Sodium content: 82mg (per 100g), 3% daily value based on a 2,000 calorie diet ✔
➢ Sugar content: 0g (per 100g) ✔

Remove chicken skin before eating. Chicken is often injected with saltwater solutions during processing (source: *Health Central*) to keep it juicy. Go for chicken not injected with fat or salt.

Always check the nutrition labels before buying and eat no more than 2 servings a day.

Chickpeas:

➢ Saturated fat content: 0.6g (per 100g) ✔
➢ Sodium content: 24mg (per 100g), 1% daily value based on a 2,000 calorie diet ✔
➢ Sugar content: 11g (per 100g) ☠

Low in saturated fat and sodium content but high in sugar. Eat in moderation. Mayo Clinic notes chickpeas as a healthy option on the DASH diet.

Chicory:

➢ Saturated fat content: 0g (per 100g) ✔
➢ Sodium content: 22mg (per 100g), less than 1% daily value based on a 2,000 calorie diet ✔
➢ Sugar content: 0.3g (per 100g) ✔

Also known as *endive*. This lovely veg is great for balancing flavors in dishes as it adds acidity and sweetness (source: *Mashed*), plus it's allowed on the DASH diet. Eat 4-5 servings of vegetables a day.

Chili pepper, red, fresh:

➢ Saturated fat content: 0g (per 100g) ✔
➢ Sodium content: 9mg (per 100g), less than 1% daily value based on a 2,000 calorie diet ✔
➢ Sugar content: 5g (per 100g) ✔

Capsaicin is the compound in chilis that gives the heat. Research has shown that this compound reduces blood pressure in rats but it hasn't yet been carried out on humans (source: *Nicswell)*.

Allowed on the DASH diet.

Chives:

➢ Saturated fat content: 0.1g (per 100g) ✔

> ➢ Sodium content: 3mg (per 100g), less than 1% daily value based on a 2,000 calorie diet ✔
> ➢ Sugar content: 1.9g (per 100g) ✔

Allowed on the DASH diet. Use chives to enhance the flavour of your dishes.

Chocolate:

> ➢ Saturated fat content: 19g (per 100g) ☹
> ➢ Sodium content: 24mg (per 100g), 1% daily value based on a 2,000 calorie diet ✔
> ➢ Sugar content: 48g (per 100g) ☹

Dark chocolate is high in flavonoids which can help lower bad cholesterol (source: *heart.org*). The American Medical Association has published a study which shows eating dark chocolate can lower blood pressure however, Alice H. Lichtenstein, the Gershoff professor of nutrition science and policy at Tufts University in Boston states:

«*While dark chocolate has more flavanols than other types of chocolate, the data to suggest there is enough to have a health effect is thin at this point.*"

Be aware of caffeine in chocolate as this may cause a spike in blood pressure.

Avoid white chocolate as it's high in saturated fat and sugar. It's not considered chocolate since it's not made of cocoa solids.

Cilantro:

➢ Saturated fat content: 0.014g (per 100g) ✓
➢ Sodium content: 46mg (per 100g), 2% daily value based on a 2,000 calorie diet ✓
➢ Sugar content: 0.87g (per 100g) ✓

Allowed on the DASH diet. Use cilantro to enhance the flavour of your dishes.

Cinnamon:

➢ Saturated fat content: 0.3g (per 100g) ✓
➢ Sodium content: 10mg (per 100g), less than 1% daily value based on a 2,000 calorie diet ✓
➢ Sugar content: 2.2g (per 100g) ✓

Allowed on the DASH diet. A lovely spice that you can add to sweet and savoury dishes. A study found consuming cinnamon short term is linked to a reduction in systolic blood pressure and diastolic blood pressure.

(source: *Akilen R, Pimlott Z, Tsiami A, Robinson N. Effect of short-term administration of cinnamon on blood pressure in patients with predi-abetes and type 2 diabetes.*)

Citrus fruits:

Lemon

➢ Saturated fat content: 0g (per 100g) ✔
➢ Sodium content: 2mg (per 100g), less than 1% daily value based on a 2,000 calorie diet ✔
➢ Sugar content: 2.5g (per 100g) ✔

Allowed on the DASH diet. Lemon juice is great for adding flavour to your dish.

Lime

➢ Saturated fat content: 0g (per 100g) ✔
➢ Sodium content: 2mg (per 100g), less than 1% daily value based on a 2,000 calorie diet ✔
➢ Sugar content: 1.7g (per 100g) ✔

Allowed on the DASH diet. Citrus fruits are full of vitamins and minerals and may even lower your blood pressure.

Cloves:

➢ Saturated fat content: 5.438g (per 100g) 💀
➢ Sodium content: 243mg (per 100g), 11% daily value based on a 2,000 calorie diet 💀
➢ Sugar content: 2.38g (per 100g) ✔

Low in sugar but thought to be high in saturated fat and sodium content. Avoid on the DASH diet.

Cocoa butter and cacao butter:

➢ Saturated fat content: 60g (per 100g) ☠
➢ Sodium content: 0mg (per 100g) ✓
➢ Sugar content: 0mg (per 100g) ✓

Cocoa has been found to reduce blood pressure however, *"long-term trials are needed to determine whether cocoa has an effect on cardiovascular events."*

(source: *Ried K, Fakler P, Stocks NP. Effect of cocoa on blood pressure. Cochrane Database Syst Rev. 2017;4(4):CD008893*)

Cocoa drinks, powder, etc:

➢ Saturated fat content: 8g (per 100g) ☠
➢ Sodium content: 21mg (per 100g), less than 1% daily value based on a 2,000 calorie diet ☠
➢ Sugar content: 1.8g (per 100g) ✓

Low in sugar but thought to be high in saturated fat and sodium content. Avoid on the DASH diet.

Coconut and coconut derivatives:

➢ Saturated fat content: 30g (per 100g) ☠
➢ Sodium content: 20mg (per 100g), less than 1% daily value based on a 2,000 calorie diet ✓
➢ Sugar content: 6g (per 100g) ☠

High in saturated fat and sugar. Avoid cooking with coconut oil, there hasn't been much research done to support the benefits of coconut oil however, it is known that drinking coconut water decreases blood pressure.

(source: *Alleyne T, Roache S, Thomas C, Shirley A. The control of hypertension by use of coconut water and mauby: two tropical food drinks. West Indian Med J. 2005*)

Coffee:

➢ Saturated fat content: 0g (per 100g) ✔
➢ Sodium content: 2mg (per 100g), less than 1% daily value based on a 2,000 calorie diet ✔
➢ Sugar content: 0g (per 100g) ✔

Allowed on the DASH diet. Go for Americano to reduce your calorie intake. Coffee lovers: do not drink too much as drinking more than four cups a day may increase your blood pressure (source: *NHS*).

Coriander:

See *cilantro*.

Cornflakes:

➢ Saturated fat content: 0.1g (per 100g) ✔
➢ Sodium content: 729mg (per 100g), 30% daily value based on a 2,000 calorie diet 😨
➢ Sugar content: 10g (per 100g) 😨

Avoid. Cornflakes may increase your risk of developing heart disease (source: *Health Day*).

Courgette:

➢ Saturated fat content: 0.1g (per 100g) ✔
➢ Sodium content: 8mg (per 100g), less than 1% daily value based on a 2,000 calorie diet ✔
➢ Sugar content: 2.5g (per 100g) ✔

Allowed on the DASH diet. You may use courgette as a base to making a healthy Bruschetta.

Crab:

➢ Saturated fat content: 0.1g (per 100g) ✔
➢ Sodium content: 1,072mg (per 100g), 44% daily value based on a 2,000 calorie diet ☠
➢ Sugar content: 0g (per 100g) ✔

High in sodium, best to avoid. Whilst crab is high in sodium, I came across sources that suggest the benefits outweigh the risks. Crabs are high in protein and low in calories.

Mayo Clinic's website features crab cakes as a sample menu created by the clinic's dieticians.

Cranberries:

➢ Saturated fat content: 0.1g (per 100g) ✔

➢ Sodium content: 3mg (per 100g), less than 1% daily value based on a 2,000 calorie diet ✓
➢ Sugar content: 65g (per 100g) 💀

Despite being high in sugar, they're full of vitamins and minerals. Cranberries are thought to boost your digestive health and promote heart health (source: *heart.org*). Avoid dried cranberries as they're full of sugar.

Cranberry juice:

➢ Saturated fat content: 0g (per 100g) ✓
➢ Sodium content: 2mg (per 100g), less than 1% daily value based on a 2,000 calorie diet ✓
➢ Sugar content: 12g (per 100g) 💀

Low in saturated fat and sodium content but high in sugar. A study found cranberry juice reduced blood pressure and lipoprotein profile although further studies are needed to verify the findings.

(source: *Richter CK, Skulas-Ray AC, Gaugler TL, Meily S, Petersen KS, Kris-Etherton PM. Effects of Cranberry Juice Supplementation on Cardiovascular Disease Risk Factors in Adults with Elevated Blood Pressure: A Randomized Controlled Trial. Nutrients. 2021 Jul 29;13(8):2618.*)

Crawfish:

➢ Saturated fat content: 0.163g (per 100g) ✓

- ➢ Sodium content: 62mg (per 100g), 3% daily value based on a 2,000 calorie diet ✔
- ➢ Sugar content: 0g (per 100g) ✔

Also known as *crayfish*. Allowed on the DASH diet.

Cream cheeses:

- ➢ Saturated fat content: 19g (per 100g) ☠
- ➢ Sodium content: 321mg (per 100g), 13% daily value based on a 2,000 calorie diet ☠
- ➢ Sugar content: 3.2g (per 100g) ✔

Low in sugar but thought to be high in saturated fat and sodium content. It's also high in calories. Avoid on the DASH diet.

If you want to enjoy cheese, go for naturally low-sodium cheese such as swiss, goat, brick ricotta and fresh mozzarella.

Cream:

- ➢ Saturated fat content: 12g (per 100g) ☠
- ➢ Sodium content: 40mg (per 100g), 1% daily value based on a 2,000 calorie diet ✔
- ➢ Sugar content: 0.1g (per 100g) ✔

Avoid cream but if you do eat it, go for low fat cream and consume in moderation. Too much saturated fat is linked to poor heart health.

Cress:

➢ Saturated fat content: 0g (per 100g) ✔
➢ Sodium content: 14mg (per 100g), less than 1% daily value based on a 2,000 calorie diet ✔
➢ Sugar content: 4.4g (per 100g) ✔

A great garnish and allowed on the DASH diet. They're full of nitrates which helps lower your blood pressure.

Cucumber:

➢ Saturated fat content: 0.034g (per 100g) ✔
➢ Sodium content: 2mg (per 100g), less than 1% daily value based on a 2,000 calorie diet ✔
➢ Sugar content: 1.67g (per 100g) ✔

Allowed on the DASH diet plus they're low in calories too. There are so many ways to include cucumber in your diet. You can eat them raw with salad or as a snack, they can be cooked or be used for smoothie. Eat 4-5 servings of vegetables a day.

Cumin:

➢ Saturated fat content: 1.5g (per 100g) 😵
➢ Sodium content: 168mg (per 100g), 7% daily value based on a 2,000 calorie diet 😵
➢ Sugar content: 2.3g (per 100g) ✔

Low in sugar but thought to be high in saturated fat and sodium content. The National Kidney Foundation's website lists cumin as allowed on this diet.

Harvard Medical School's website suggests making a vegetarian chilli with cumin and other ingredients such as beans, onions, canned tomatoes, minced garlic and chilli powder.

Curry:

➢ Saturated fat content: 2.2g (per 100g) ☠
➢ Sodium content: 52mg (per 100g), 2% daily value based on a 2,000 calorie diet ✓
➢ Sugar content: 2.8g (per 100g) ✓

Curries are usually made of turmeric, coriander, cumin, ginger, chilli powder and pepper. WebMD noted a study found *"people who eat more curry powder are less likely to have high blood pressure"*.

Why not try chickpea curry? Eating Well's website features a quick and healthy recipe.

Dates:

➢ Saturated fat content: 0.032g (per 100g) ✓
➢ Sodium content: 0mg (per 100g) ✓
➢ Sugar content: 63.35g (per 100g) ☠

(source: *Fatsecret Platform API*)

Low in saturated fat and sodium content but high in sugar. The sugar in dates are natural and several sources suggest dates are allowed on the DASH diet.

Dextrose:

➤ Saturated fat content: 0g (per 100g) ✔
➤ Sodium content: N/A (per 100g) ✔
➤ Sugar content: 92.7g (per 100g) 😨

Sugar from corn. There isn't any benefit from eating sugar. The American Heart Association recommends no more than 24g of sugar for women and no more than 36g of sugar per day for men. 100g of dextrose exceeds the sugar recommendations per day. Avoid.

Dill:

➤ Saturated fat content: 0.1g (per 100g) ✔
➤ Sodium content: 61mg (per 100g), 2% daily value based on a 2,000 calorie diet ✔
➤ Sugar content: N/A (per 100g) ✔

Allowed on the DASH diet. Dill is a fragrant spice that's great for freshening up your dishes.

Dragon fruit:

➤ Saturated fat content: N/A (1 fruit) ✔
➤ Sodium content: N/A (1 fruit) ✔
➤ Sugar content: 8g (1 fruit) 😨

Often known as *white-fleshed pitahaya*. Dragon fruits are an excellent source of fiber, magnesium, iron, vitamin C, carotenoids and lycopene. Low in saturated fat and sodium content but high in sugar. Eat in moderation.

Dried fruit:

➤ Saturated fat content: 0.7g (per 100g) ✓
➤ Sodium content: 403mg (per 100g), 16% daily value based on a 2,000 calorie diet 😟
➤ Sugar content: 58g (per 100g) 😟

These included raisins, dates, prunes, apricots to name a few. Dried fruits are high in calories. Best to avoid although I recommend you check the nutritional values for each dried fruit. Dates are thought to be the healthier dried fruit. See *Dates* above.

Dried meat:

➤ Saturated fat content: 1.6g (per 100g) 😟
➤ Sodium content: 950mg (per 100g), 39% daily value based on a 2,000 calorie diet 😟
➤ Sugar content: 0g (per 100g) ✓

Low in sugar but thought to be high in saturated fat and sodium content. Dried meat is a highly processed food. Avoid on the DASH diet.

Dry-cured meats:
Beef

- ➢ Saturated fat content: 0.95g (per 100g) ✔
- ➢ Sodium content: 2,790mg (per 100g), 121% daily value based on a 2,000 calorie diet 💀
- ➢ Sugar content: 2.45g (per 100g) ✔

Pork

- ➢ Saturated fat content: 1g (per 100g) ✔
- ➢ Sodium content: 320mg (per 100g), 14% daily value based on a 2,000 calorie diet 💀
- ➢ Sugar content: 10g (per 100g) 💀

These are meats that have been salted, dried and aged to preserve them from harmful bacteria. They contain unhealthy amounts of sodium on the DASH diet. Avoid.

Duck:

- ➢ Saturated fat content: 10g (per 100g) 💀
- ➢ Sodium content: 59mg (per 100g), 2% daily value based on a 2,000 calorie diet ✔
- ➢ Sugar content: 0g (per 100g) ✔

Do not eat the skin and avoid crispy duck. SF Gate recommends going for baked, roasted or braised duck. Limit to one serving a day without the skin.

Egg white:

➤ Saturated fat content: 0g (per 100g) ✓
➤ Sodium content: 166mg (per 100g), 6% daily value based on a 2,000 calorie diet 💀
➤ Sugar content: 0.7g (per 100g) ✓

Eggs are high in cholesterol so limit consumption (source: *Harvard Medical School*) however, a study found eggs have no significant effect on blood pressure.

(source: *Kolahdouz-Mohammadi R, Malekahmadi M, Clayton ZS, et al. Effect of Egg Consumption on Blood Pressure: a Systematic Review and Meta-analysis of Randomized Clinical Trials.*)

Egg yolk:

➤ Saturated fat content: 10g (per 100g) 💀
➤ Sodium content: 48mg (per 100g), 2% daily value based on a 2,000 calorie diet ✓
➤ Sugar content: 0.6g (per 100g) ✓

Limit egg yolk intake to no more than four a week as eggs are high in cholesterol (source: *Harvard Medical School*).

Elderflower cordial:

➤ Saturated fat content: 0g (per 25ml) ✓
➤ Sodium content: N/A (per 25ml) ✓
➤ Sugar content: 5.6g (per 25ml) 💀

Low in saturated fat and sodium content but high in sugar. A study on mice found elderflower lowered systolic blood pressure by five percent and diastolic blood pressure by two and half percent. More research is needed to back this up (source: *Smart Supplements Guide*).

Endive:

➢ Saturated fat content: 0g (per 100g) ✓
➢ Sodium content: 22mg (per 100g), less than 1% daily value based on a 2,000 calorie diet ✓
➢ Sugar content: 0.3g (per 100g) ✓

Allowed on the DASH diet. Endive is low in calories and helps regulate blood sugar levels. It's high in potassium which is great for your heart health.

Espresso:

➢ Saturated fat content: 0.1g (per 100g) ✓
➢ Sodium content: 14mg (per 100g), less than 1% daily value based on a 2,000 calorie diet ✓
➢ Sugar content: 0g (per 100g) ✓

Allowed on the DASH diet. Espresso is thought to contain more caffeine than coffee. Watch out for your caffeine intake. Drinking more than four cups a day may increase your blood pressure (source: *NHS).*

Fennel:

➢ Saturated fat content: 0.2g (per 100g) ✔
➢ Sodium content: 52mg (per 100g), 2% daily value based on a 2,000 calorie diet ✔
➢ Sugar content: N/A (per 100g) ✔

Allowed on the DASH diet. Fennel contains nitrates which are thought to help lower blood pressure. Eat 4-5 servings of vegetables a day.

Fenugreek:

➢ Saturated fat content: 1.5g (per 100g) ☹
➢ Sodium content: 0mg (per 100g) ✔
➢ Sugar content: N/A (per 100g) ✔

A herb that has many health benefits such as reducing the risk of cancer, diabetes, obesity, high blood pressure and inflammation to name a few (source: *Medical News Today*). Fenugreek is thought to lower blood pressure and blood sugar. A source suggests to not consume fenugreek every day.

Feta cheese:

➢ Saturated fat content: 15g (per 100g) ☹
➢ Sodium content: 1,116mg (per 100g), 46% daily value based on a 2,000 calorie diet ☹
➢ Sugar content: 4.1g (per 100g) ✔

Low in sugar but thought to be high in saturated fat and sodium content. Limit cheese intake if you're following the DASH diet but if you must eat cheese, go for low-fat cheese such as feta.

Figs (fresh or dried):

➤ Saturated fat content: 0.06g (per 100g) ✔
➤ Sodium content: 1mg (per 100g), less than 1% daily value based on a 2,000 calorie diet ✔
➤ Sugar content: 16.26g (per 100g) ☻

Low in saturated fat and sodium content but high in sugar. Eat in moderation.

Fish:

➤ Saturated fat content: 2.5g (per 100g) ☻
➤ Sodium content: 61mg (per 100g), 2% daily value based on a 2,000 calorie diet ✔
➤ Sugar content: N/A (per 100g) ✔

Avoided salted fish. Fresh fish is acceptable. If the fish is canned or frozen, ensure it is low-sodium as salt is often added to preserve the fish for longer. *The DASH Diet for Hypertension by Mark Jenkins and Thomas J. Moore* suggests all fish are naturally low in saturated fat. They recommend choosing fish over chicken or beef.

Flaxseed (linseed):

➤ Saturated fat content: 3.7g (per 100g) ☻

➢ Sodium content: 30mg (per 100g), 1% daily value based on a 2,000 calorie diet ✔
➢ Sugar content: 1.6g (per 100g) ✔

Ensure you eat no more than 4-5 servings a week. Eating Well's website notes flaxseeds as part of the DASH diet and a heart-healthy lifestyle.

Fructose (fruit sugar):

➢ Saturated fat content: 0g (per 100g) ✔
➢ Sodium content: 12mg (per 100g), 1% daily value based on a 2,000 calorie diet ✔
➢ Sugar content: 92.7g (per 100g) ☹

According to the RDH (Registered Dental Hygienists), there is no biological need for fructose. RDH lists the negative health implications of consuming fructose such as the increase risk of obesity and type 2 diabetes to name a few.

Due to the potential negative health implications, this guide recommends avoiding processed fructose where possible.

Game (meat):

➢ Saturated fat content: 1g (per 100g) ✔
➢ Sodium content: 51mg (per 100g), 2% daily value based on a 2,000 calorie diet ✔
➢ Sugar content: 0g (per 100g) ✔

(source: *Nutrition Value*)

The DASH diet recommends lean meat if you have to eat meat. Game is lean which means it's high in protein and low in fat. Allowed on the DASH diet. Eat no more than 2 servings a day.

Garlic:

➢ Saturated fat content: 0.089g (per 100g) ✓
➢ Sodium content: 17mg (per 100g), 1% daily value based on a 2,000 calorie diet ✓
➢ Sugar content: 1g (per 100g) ✓

Allowed on the DASH diet. PubMed have published a study confirming garlic helps reduce blood pressure.

(source: *Ried K, Frank OR, Stocks NP, Fakler P, Sullivan T. Effect of garlic on blood pressure: a systematic review and meta-analysis. BMC Cardiovasc Disord*)

Ginger:

➢ Saturated fat content: 0.2g (per 100g) ✓
➢ Sodium content: 13mg (per 100g), less than 1% daily value based on a 2,000 calorie diet ✓
➢ Sugar content: 1.7g (per 100g) ✓

Allowed on the DASH diet. Ginger has been shown to reduce blood pressure. Add this spice to brighten up your dish.

Goat's milk:

➤ Saturated fat content: 2.7g (per 100g) 😟
➤ Sodium content: 50mg (per 100g), 2% daily value based on a 2,000 calorie diet ✔
➤ Sugar content: 4.5g (per 100g) ✔

A study found goat's milk lowers blood pressure and prevents hypertension in sedentary women. This is a great alternative to cow's milk as goat's milk is thought to be naturally lower in cholesterol. Go for low-fat goat's milk.

(Source: *https://www.atlantis-press.com/proceedings/phico-16/25875903*)

Goji berry:

➤ Saturated fat content: 0.4g (per 100g) ✔
➤ Sodium content: 298mg (per 100g), 13% daily value based on a 2,000 calorie diet 😟
➤ Sugar content: 46g (per 100g) 😟

(source: *Nutrition Value*)

A few sources point to goji berries lowering blood pressure however, be aware that these berries may react to certain medications such as blood thinners, diabetes and blood pressure medication (source: *Healthline*). They're also higher in sodium and sugar content than other berries so eat in moderation.

Goose (organic, freshly cooked):

➢ Saturated fat content: 4.56g (per 100g) ☻
➢ Sodium content: 76mg (per 100g), 3% daily value based on a 2,000 calorie diet ✔
➢ Sugar content: N/A (per 100g) ✔

One source notes the high nutrition content in goose meat but doesn't recommend it for people with high blood pressure.

The legs and skin of geese have the highest amount of fat content so remove these before eating. Go for the breast meat as this has less fat (source: *Health and Social Services, Government of Northwest Territories*).

Gooseberry, gooseberries:

➢ Saturated fat content: 0.038g (per 100g) ✔
➢ Sodium content: 1mg (per 100g), less than 1% daily value based on a 2,000 calorie diet ✔
➢ Sugar content: N/A (per 100g) ✔

A soft fruit that's allowed on the DASH diet. According to Eat Delights' blog, gooseberries tastes similar to strawberries, apples and grapes. What an interesting combination.

Gouda cheese:

➢ Saturated fat content: 18g (per 100g) ☻

- ➢ Sodium content: 819mg (per 100g), 34% daily value based on a 2,000 calorie diet 😕
- ➢ Sugar content: 2.2g (per 100g) ✔

Low in sugar but thought to be high in saturated fat and sodium content. Avoid on the DASH diet. If you want to eat cheese, Livestrong's website suggests going for Swiss, Feta or Parmesan.

Grapefruit:

- ➢ Saturated fat content: 0g (per 100g) ✔
- ➢ Sodium content: 0mg (per 100g) ✔
- ➢ Sugar content: 7g (per 100g) 😕

Low in saturated fat and sodium content but high in sugar. Eat in moderation. Watch out if you're taking medication as grapefruit may interfere with some blood pressure medication (source: *Harvard Health*).

Grapes:

- ➢ Saturated fat content: 0.1g (per 100g) ✔
- ➢ Sodium content: 2mg (per 100g), less than 1% daily value based on a 2,000 calorie diet ✔
- ➢ Sugar content: 16g (per 100g) 😕

Low in saturated fat and sodium content but high in sugar. Limit grapes in your meal plan.

Green beans – see "beans"

➢ Saturated fat content: 0g (per 100g) ✔
➢ Sodium content: 6mg (per 100g), less than 1% daily value based on a 2,000 calorie diet ✔
➢ Sugar content: N/A (per 100g) ✔

Allowed on the DASH diet. Try roasting green beans with herbs, garlic and olive oil — it tastes delicious. Eat 4-5 servings of vegetables a day.

Green peas:

➢ Saturated fat content: 0.1g (per 100g) ✔
➢ Sodium content: 5mg (per 100g), less than 1% daily value based on a 2,000 calorie diet ✔
➢ Sugar content: 6g (per 100g) ☠

Low in saturated fat and sodium content but high in sugar. Multiple sources allow green peas on the DASH diet.

Green tea:

➢ Saturated fat content: 0.002g (per 100g) ✔
➢ Sodium content: 1mg (per 100g), less than 1% daily value based on a 2,000 calorie diet ✔
➢ Sugar content: 0g (per 100g) ✔

Allowed on the DASH diet. The flavonoids in green tea have been shown to lower LDL cholesterol levels (source: *Dietician UK*).

Guava:

- ➢ Saturated fat content: 0.3g (per 100g) ✓
- ➢ Sodium content: 2mg (per 100g), less than 1% daily value based on a 2,000 calorie diet ✓
- ➢ Sugar content: 9g (per 100g) ☹

Low in saturated fat and sodium content but high in sugar. Guava is high in potassium and one study found *"120 people who ate guava before each meal for 12 weeks saw a reduction in total cholesterol and blood pressure, and experienced an increase in good (HDL) cholesterol."*

(source: *Singh RB, Rastogi SS, Singh R, Ghosh S, Niaz MA. Effects of guava intake on serum total and high-density lipoprotein cholesterol levels and on systemic blood pressure. Am J Cardiol.*)

Ham (dried, cured):

- ➢ Saturated fat content: 1.8g (per 100g) ☹
- ➢ Sodium content: 1,203mg (per 100g), 50% daily value based on a 2,000 calorie diet ☹
- ➢ Sugar content: 0g (per 100g) ✓

Low in sugar but thought to be high in saturated fat and sodium content. Ham is processed red meat. The American Institute of Cancer Research reported a link between cancer and processed meat. Avoid on the DASH diet.

Hazelnut:

➤ Saturated fat content: 4.5g (per 100g) 💀
➤ Sodium content: 0mg (per 100g) ✔
➤ Sugar content: 4.3g (per 100g) ✔

Ensure you eat no more than 4-5 servings a week and go for unsalted nuts. Eating Well's website notes hazelnuts as part of the DASH diet and a heart-healthy lifestyle.

Hemp seeds (Cannabis sativa):

➤ Saturated fat content: 4.6g (per 100g) 💀
➤ Sodium content: 5mg (per 100g), less than 1% daily value based on a 2,000 calorie diet ✔
➤ Sugar content: 1.5g (per 100g) ✔

(source: *Nutrition Value*)

They're full of omega-3 fatty acids which are needed for a healthy heart. Ensure you eat no more than 4-5 servings a week.

Herbal tea:

➤ Saturated fat content: 0.3g (per 100g) ✔
➤ Sodium content: 3mg (per 100g), less than 1% daily value based on a 2,000 calorie diet ✔
➤ Sugar content: 6g (per 100g) 💀

Low in saturated fat and sodium content but high in sugar. Check the nutrition labels and make sure the herbal tea is unsweetened. Drink in moderation.

Honey:

- ➢ Saturated fat content: 0g (per 100g) ✔
- ➢ Sodium content: 4mg (per 100g), less than 1% daily value based on a 2,000 calorie diet ✔
- ➢ Sugar content: 82g (per 100g) 😧

Low in saturated fat and sodium content but high in sugar. Avoid adding sugar to your diet even if it's honey. Eat in moderation.

Horseradish:

- ➢ Saturated fat content: 0.09g (per 100g) ✔
- ➢ Sodium content: 314mg (per 100g), 14% daily value based on a 2,000 calorie diet 😧
- ➢ Sugar content: 7.99g (per 100g) 😧

(source: *Fatsecret Platform API*)

Whilst this root veg is thought to help reduce inflammation, fight cell damage and improve respiratory health (source: *WebMD*), it's relatively high in sodium and sugar. Limit consumption.

Juniper berries:

- ➢ Saturated fat content: 0g (per 100g) ✔
- ➢ Sodium content: N/A (per 100g) ✔
- ➢ Sugar content: 4.2g (per 100g) ✔

(source: *Nutrition Value*)

Allowed on the DASH diet. They're packed full of anti-oxidants too.

Kale:

➢ Saturated fat content: 0.091g (per 100g) ✔
➢ Sodium content: 43mg (per 100g), 2% daily value based on a 2,000 calorie diet ✔
➢ Sugar content: N/A (per 100g) ✔

Allowed on the DASH diet. Kale is thought to help lower blood pressure naturally.

Have you tried kale chips? They're a great crispy snack and a healthy alternative to potato chips. Consume 4-5 servings of vegetables a day.

Kefir:

➢ Saturated fat content: 1.669g (per 100g) ☹
➢ Sodium content: 41mg (per 100g), 2% daily value based on a 2,000 calorie diet ✔
➢ Sugar content: 4.88g (per 100g) ✔

Very high in fat — best to avoid however, a source suggests drinking kefir may have a positive effect on blood pressure.

A study has shown traditional kefir may help control blood cholesterol levels however, more studies need to be carried out as traditional kefir may differ from commercial kefir.

(source: *https://clinicaltrials.gov/ct2/show/NCT04247139*)

Kelp:

➢ Saturated fat content: 0.2g (per 100g) ✓
➢ Sodium content: 233mg (per 100g), 10% daily value based on a 2,000 calorie diet 💀
➢ Sugar content: 0.6g (per 100g) ✓

(source: *Nutrition Value*)

Winchester Hospital notes kelp has been used to "*promote weight loss and lower blood pressure*" but there isn't enough study to demonstrate the benefits of kelp in treating health problems. Watch the sodium content.

Kiwi:

➢ Saturated fat content: 0g (per 100g) ✓
➢ Sodium content: 3mg (per 100g), less than 1% daily value based on a 2,000 calorie diet ✓
➢ Sugar content: 9g (per 100g) 💀

Low in saturated fat and sodium content but high in sugar. Kiwis are thought to be rich in vitamin C which may improve blood pressure. A study on men and women with moderately elevated blood pressure found:

"Intake of three kiwifruits was associated with lower systolic and diastolic 24-h BP compared with one apple a day."

(source: *Svendsen M, Tonstad S, Heggen E, Pedersen TR, Seljeflot I, Bøhn SK, Bastani NE, Blomhoff R, Holme IM, Klemsdal TO. The effect of kiwifruit consumption on blood pressure in subjects with moderately elevated blood pressure: a randomized, controlled study. Blood Press. 2015*)

Kohlrabi:

➤ Saturated fat content: 0g (per 100g) ✔
➤ Sodium content: 20mg (per 100g), less than 1% daily value based on a 2,000 calorie diet ✔
➤ Sugar content: 2.6g (per 100g) ✔

Also known as *German turnip*. Similar to cabbage, Cook For Your Life's blog notes kohlrabi may be eaten raw, steamed or blanched plus it's allowed on the DASH diet. Eat 4-5 servings of vegetables a day.

Lamb:

➤ Saturated fat content: 9g (per 100g), 45% daily value based on a 2,000 calorie diet ☠
➤ Sodium content: 72mg (per 100g), 3% daily value based on a 2,000 calorie diet ✔
➤ Sugar content: 0g (per 100g) ✔

High in fat. Limit consumption of red meat such as lamb.

Lamb's lettuce, corn salad:

➤ Saturated fat content: 1g (per 100g) ✔
➤ Sodium content: 177.5mg (per 100g), 7% daily value based on a 2,000 calorie diet ☻
➤ Sugar content: 4g (per 100g) ✔

(source: *Nutritionix*)

Corn salad is usually made with corn kernels, tomatoes, cucumbers, feta and herbs. It's thought to be allowed on the DASH diet as it's high in potassium which protects against cardiovascular disease.

It's great for warm weather too. Why not take this healthy dish with you on your next picnic?

Lard:

➤ Saturated fat content: 32g (per 100g) ☻
➤ Sodium content: 27mg (per 100g), 1% daily value based on a 2,000 calorie diet ✔
➤ Sugar content: 0g (per 100g) ✔

Lard is a source of fat — watch your intake as too much fat will raise your blood pressure. Interesting fact: lard has 20% less saturated fat than butter (source: *Supermarket Guru*). Other sources suggest cooking with lard instead of butter.

Leek:

➢ Saturated fat content: 0g (per 100g) ✔
➢ Sodium content: 20mg (per 100g), less than 1% daily value based on a 2,000 calorie diet ✔
➢ Sugar content: 3.9g (per 100g) ✔

Low in calories and allowed on the DASH diet. Eat 4-5 servings of vegetables a day.

Lemon:

➢ Saturated fat content: 0g (per 100g) ✔
➢ Sodium content: 2mg (per 100g), less than 1% daily value based on a 2,000 calorie diet ✔
➢ Sugar content: 2.5g (per 100g) ✔

Allowed on the DASH diet. Lemon juice is great for adding flavour to your dish.

Lentils:

➢ Saturated fat content: 0.1g (per 100g) ✔
➢ Sodium content: 2mg (per 100g), less than 1% daily value based on a 2,000 calorie diet ✔
➢ Sugar content: 1.8g (per 100g) ✔

Allowed on the DASH diet. A daily cup of lentils is thought to "*keep your blood pressure in check*" (source: *WebMD*).

Lettuce:

➤ Saturated fat content: 0g (per 100g) ✔
➤ Sodium content: 28mg (per 100g), 1% daily value based on a 2,000 calorie diet ✔
➤ Sugar content: 0.8g (per 100g) ✔

Allowed on the DASH diet. Eat 4-5 servings of vegetables a day.

Lime:

➤ Saturated fat content: 0g (per 100g) ✔
➤ Sodium content: 2mg (per 100g), less than 1% daily value based on a 2,000 calorie diet ✔
➤ Sugar content: 1.7g (per 100g) ✔

Allowed on the DASH diet. Citrus fruits are full of vitamins and minerals and may even lower your blood pressure.

Liquor:

➤ Saturated fat content: 0g (per 100g) ✔
➤ Sodium content: 1mg (per 100g), less than 1% daily value based on a 2,000 calorie diet ✔
➤ Sugar content: 0g (per 100g) ✔

Avoid sweetened liquor. Liquor is allowed on the DASH diet but many sources advise drinking alcohol sparingly.

Liquorice:

➤ Saturated fat content: 1.3g (per 100g) 😖

- Sodium content: 162mg (per 100g), 7% daily value based on a 2,000 calorie diet 🤔
- Sugar content: 40g (per 100g) 🤔

(source: *Nutrition Value*)

Avoid. The NHS notes:

"Eating more than 57g (2 ounces) of black liquorice a day for at least 2 weeks could lead to potentially serious health problems, such as an increase in blood pressure and an irregular heart rhythm (arrhythmia)."

Lobster:

- Saturated fat content: 0.106g (per 100g) ✔
- Sodium content: 700mg (per 100g), 30% daily value based on a 2,000 calorie diet 🤔
- Sugar content: 0g (per 100g) ✔

(source: *Fatsecret Platform API*)

Watch the sodium here. Several sources seem to suggest lobster is allowed on the DASH diet. Avoid serving lobster with butter and eat in moderation.

Loganberry:

- Saturated fat content: 0.3g (per 100g) ✔

➤ Sodium content: 1mg (per 100g), less than 1% daily value based on a 2,000 calorie diet ✔
➤ Sugar content: 7.7g (per 100g) ☠

(source: *Nutrition Value*)

Low in saturated fat and sodium content but high in sugar. Eat in moderation.

Lychee:

➤ Saturated fat content: 0.1g (per 100g) ✔
➤ Sodium content: 1mg (per 100g), less than 1% daily value based on a 2,000 calorie diet ✔
➤ Sugar content: 15g (per 100g) ☠

Low in saturated fat and sodium content but high in sugar. It's thought to contain potassium which helps to maintain blood pressure. Eat in moderation.

Macadamia:

➤ Saturated fat content: 12g (per 100g) ☠
➤ Sodium content: 5 mg (per 100g), less than 1% daily value based on a 2,000 calorie diet ✔
➤ Sugar content: 4.6g (per 100g) ✔

Although macadamia nuts are high in saturated fats, like many nuts they are rich in nutrients and anti-oxidants. Due to this, macadamia nuts can be included in the DASH diet in moderation.

Malt:

➢ Saturated fat content: 1.9g (per 100g) 💀
➢ Sodium content: 60mg (per 100g), 2% daily value based on a 2,000 calorie diet ✔
➢ Sugar content: 7g (per 100g) 💀

Malt is a cereal grain that has been dried in a process called malting. Malt is often used in making beer, liquor, baked goods and desserts (source: *Food52*). Limit your intake of malt as it is higher in saturated fat and sugars.

Malt extract:

➢ Saturated fat content: <0.1g (per 100g) ✔
➢ Sodium content: Not specified
➢ Sugar content: 55.2g (per 100g) 💀

(source: *Grape Tree*)

Malt may be further processed to form malt extract (source: *Briess*). It's thought to be high in antioxidants. It's thought to be high in sugar so best to avoid.

Maltodextrin:

➢ Saturated fat content: 0g (per 100g) ✔
➢ Sodium content: 0g (per 100g), 0% of daily value based on a 2,000 calorie diet ✔
➢ Sugar content: 95.09g (per 100g) 💀

A highly processed form of carbohydrate that's extracted from corn, rice, potato and other plants. It's commonly found in artificial sweeteners, yogurt, beer, baked goods and nutrition bars to name a few (source: *Medicine Net*). As it's a powder typically found in processed foods, it's best to avoid.

Mandarin orange:

➤ Saturated fat content: 0g (per 100g) ✔
➤ Sodium content: 2 mg (per 100g), less than 1% daily value based on a 2,000 calorie diet ✔
➤ Sugar content: 11g (per 100g) ☹

Although mandarin oranges are high in sugar, they have many health benefits that may make them worthwhile to include in your diet. Mandarin oranges are loaded with fiber and potassium, both of which help to lower blood pressure (source: *WebMD*).

Mango:

➤ Saturated fat content: 0.1g (per 100g) ✔
➤ Sodium content: 1 mg (per 100g), less than 1% daily value based on a 2,000 calorie diet ✔
➤ Sugar content: 14g (per 100g) ☹

Mangoes are a higher sugar fruit, but can be consumed in moderation as part of a healthy diet.

Maple syrup:

➤ Saturated fat content: 0g (per 100g) ✔

➢ Sodium content: 12mg (per 100g), less than 1% daily value based on a 2,000 calorie diet ✔
➢ Sugar content: 68g (per 100g) 😮

Although it is high in sugar, some recommend the DASH diet to include real maple syrup as a healthy sweet treat replacement. (Source: *Winchester Hospital*)

Margarine:

➢ Saturated fat content: 15g (per 100g) 😮
➢ Sodium content: 2mg (per 100g), less than 1% daily value based on a 2,000 calorie diet ✔
➢ Sugar content: 0g ✔

Margarine is typically limited in the DASH diet due to its high saturated fat content.

Marrow:

Bone marrow:

➢ Saturated fat content: 84.4g (per 100g) 😮
➢ Sodium content: N/A
➢ Sugar content: N/A

(source: *Fatsecret Platform API*)

Vegetable marrow:

➢ Saturated fat content: 0.5g (per 100g) ✔

- ➤ Sodium content: N/A
- ➤ Sugar content: N/A

The sodium and sugar content of marrow is unknown. Avoid bone marrow as this is thought to be high in saturated fat content and high in calories.

Mascarpone cheese:

- ➤ Saturated fat content: 30g (per 100g) 🫣
- ➤ Sodium content: 33mg (per 100g), 2% daily value based on a 2,000 calorie diet ✔
- ➤ Sugar content: 3.3g (per 100g) ✔

(source: Eat This Much)

Mascarpone cheese is high in saturated fat, so try to avoid on the DASH diet.

Mate tea:

- ➤ Saturated fat content: 0g (per tea bag, 3g) ✔
- ➤ Sodium content: 0mg (per tea bag, 3g) ✔
- ➤ Sugar content: 0g (per tea bag, 3g) ✔

Mate tea is thought to help with a number of conditions such as headaches and depression (source: *Mayo Clinic*). It's high in antioxidants and a source of caffeine. Watch your intake as too much caffeine is thought to increase blood pressure.

Melon:

➢ Saturated fat content: 0.1g (per 100g) ✔
➢ Sodium content: 16mg (per 100g), less than 1% daily value based on a 2,000 calorie diet ✔
➢ Sugar content: 8g (per 100g) 💀

Fruits like melon can be eaten on the DASH diet to replace more unhealthy sweets. Try a fruit cup to appease your sweet tooth.

Milk:

➢ Saturated fat content: 0.6g (per 100g) ✔
➢ Sodium content: 44 mg (per 100g), 1% daily value based on a 2,000 calorie diet ✔
➢ Sugar content: 5g (per 100g) ✔

Allowed on the DASH diet. Dairy is a great source of protein and calcium. Opt for fat-free or low-fat milk for the best DASH diet choice (source: *Winchester Hospital*).

Millet:

➢ Saturated fat content: 0.5g (per 100g) ✔
➢ Sodium content: 4 mg (per 100g), less than 1% daily value based on a 2,000 calorie diet ✔
➢ Sugar content: 1.7g (per 100g) ✔

Allowed on the DASH diet. Millet is a healthy grain option to include in your diet.

Minced meat:

➢ Saturated fat content: 11g (per 100g) ☠
➢ Sodium content: 67mg (per 100g), 2% daily value based on a 2,000 calorie diet ✔
➢ Sugar content: 0g (per 100g) ✔

Minced meat is high in saturated fat. Try to avoid on the DASH diet.

Mint:

➢ Saturated fat content: 0.2g (per 100g) ✔
➢ Sodium content: 31 mg (per 100mg), 1% daily value based on a 2,000 calorie diet ✔
➢ Sugar content: 0g (per 100g) ✔

Allowed on the DASH diet. Use mint to spruce up dishes, or drink it as a tea.

Morel mushrooms:

➢ Saturated fat content: 0.1g (per 100g) ✔
➢ Sodium content: 21mg (per 100g) 1% daily value based on a 2,000 calorie diet ✔
➢ Sugar content: 0.6g (per 100g) ✔

(source: *Nutrition Value*)

Allowed on the DASH diet. Mushrooms are a versatile vegetable that can go with dozens of meals. Use spices to add flavor.

Morello cherries, sour cherries:

➢ Saturated fat content: 0g (per 100g) ✔
➢ Sodium content: 7.4mg (per 100g), 1% daily value based on a 2,000 calorie diet ✔
➢ Sugar content: 8.49g (per 100g) 😯

(source: *Eat This Much*)

Morello cherries are tart, sour cherries that are most often consumed dried, frozen, or juiced. Morello cherries contain 20 times more vitamin A than sweet cherries (source: *Healthline*).

Mozzarella cheese:

➢ Saturated fat content: 11g (per 100g) 😯
➢ Sodium content: 16 mg (per 100g), less than 1% daily value based on a 2,000 calorie diet ✔
➢ Sugar content: 1.2g (per 100g) ✔

Mozzarella cheese is high in saturated fat, so try to limit or avoid on the DASH diet.

Mulberry:

➢ Saturated fat content: 0g (per 100g) ✔
➢ Sodium content: 10 mg (per 100g), less than 1% daily value based on a 2,000 calorie diet ✔
➢ Sugar content: 8g 😯

Mulberries contain loads of heart-healthy antioxidants. Although they have a higher sugar content, mulberries can be part of a healthy diet in moderation.

Mungbeans (germinated, sprouting):

➢ Saturated fat content: 0.3g (per 100g) ✔
➢ Sodium content: 15 mg (per 100g), less than 1% daily value based on a 2,000 calorie diet ✔
➢ Sugar content: 7g (per 100g) ☹

Mung beans are part of the legume family. Packed with protein, fiber, and antioxidants, mung beans can be a great addition to a healthy diet (source: *Holland and Barrett*).

Mushrooms, different types:

➢ Saturated fat content: 0.1g (per 100g) ✔
➢ Sodium content: 5 mg (per 100g), less than 1% daily value based on a 2,000 calorie diet ✔
➢ Sugar content: 2g (per 100g) ✔

Allowed on the DASH diet. Mushrooms are a versatile food that can be incorporated into loads of different dishes.

Mustard and mustard seeds:

➢ Saturated fat content: 0.2g (per 100g) ✔
➢ Sodium content: 1,135mg (per 100g), 47% daily value based on a 2,000 calorie diet ☹
➢ Sugar content: 0.9g (per 100g) ✔

Mustard is high in sodium. Try to avoid or limit on the DASH diet.

Napa cabbage:

➢ Saturated fat content: 0g (per 100g) ✔
➢ Sodium content: 11mg (per 100g), less than 1% daily value based on a 2,000 calorie diet ✔
➢ Sugar content: 0g (per 100g) ✔

Allowed on the DASH diet. Napa cabbage is a type of Chinese cabbage often used in dishes such as stir fry.

Nectarine:

➢ Saturated fat content: 0g (per 100g) ✔
➢ Sodium content: 0mg (per 100g), 0% daily value based on a 2,000 calorie diet ✔
➢ Sugar content: 8g (per 100g) 💀

Nectarines are high in sugar but can be included as part of a healthy diet in moderation.

Nettle tea:

➢ Saturated fat content: 0g (per 100g) ✔
➢ Sodium content: 0g (per 100g), 0% daily value based on a 2,000 calorie diet ✔
➢ Sugar content: 0g (per 100g) ✔

Nettle tea is made from infusing a stinging nettle plant in hot water. Nettle tea is rich in antioxidants (source: *Medical News Today*).

Nori seaweed:

➤ Saturated fat content: 0.1g (per 100g) ✔
➤ Sodium content: 48mg (per 100g), 2% daily value based on a 2,000 calorie diet ✔
➤ Sugar content: 0.5g (per 100g) ✔

Allowed on the DASH diet. Nori seaweed boasts many health benefits such as supporting heart health, boosting the immune system, and balancing blood sugar levels (source: *BBC Good Food*).

Nutmeg:

➤ Saturated fat content: 26g (per 100g) ☠
➤ Sodium content: 16 mg (per 100g), less than 1% daily value based on a 2,000 calorie diet ✔
➤ Sugar content: 28g (per 100g) ✔

Avoid eating large amounts of nutmeg as it is high in saturated fat.

Nuts: (see individual nuts for more details)

➤ Saturated fat content: 9g (per 100g) ☠
➤ Sodium content: 273mg (per 100g), 11% daily value based on a 2,000 calorie diet ✔
➤ Sugar content: 4.2 g (per 100g) ✔

Nuts are a vital part of the DASH diet. They add protein and healthy fat to your diet. They can be high in saturated fat, so be sure to eat in moderation.

Oats:

➢ Saturated fat content: 0.2g (per 100g) ✔
➢ Sodium content: 49mg (per 100g), 2% daily value based on a 2,000 calorie diet ✔
➢ Sugar content: 0.5g (per 100g) ✔

Allowed on the DASH diet. Incorporate oats into your diet to add some healthy whole grains.

Olive oil:

➢ Saturated fat content: 14g (per 100g) 💀
➢ Sodium content: 2mg (per 100g), less than 1% daily value based on a 2,000 calorie diet ✔
➢ Sugar content: 0g (per 100g) ✔

Olive oil is a healthy source of fat in the DASH diet. Consume in moderation.

Olives (black):

➢ Saturated fat content: 1.2g (per 100g) 💀
➢ Sodium content: 880mg (per 100g), 38% daily value based on a 2,000 calorie diet 💀
➢ Sugar content: 0g (per 100g)

(source: *Fatsecret Platform API*)

Olives are high in saturated fat and sodium. Limit or avoid on the DASH diet.

Onion:

➢ Saturated fat content: 0g (per 100g) ✔
➢ Sodium content: 4mg (per 100g), less than 1% daily value based on a 2,000 calorie diet ✔
➢ Sugar content: 4.2g (per 100g) ✔

Allowed on the DASH diet. Onions are a great way to enhance flavor without adding extra salt to a meal.

Orange:

➢ Saturated fat content: 0g (per 100g) ✔
➢ Sodium content: 0g (per 100g), 0% daily value based on a 2,000 calorie diet ✔
➢ Sugar content: 9g (per 100g) 💀

Oranges are high in sugar, but can be included in moderation on the DASH diet.

Oregano:

➢ Saturated fat content: 2.66g (per 100g) 💀
➢ Sodium content: 15mg (per 100g), 1% daily value based on a 2,000 calorie diet ✔
➢ Sugar content: 4g (per 100g) ✔

Oregano can be used in moderation to add flavor to dishes.

Ostrich:

➢ Saturated fat content: 1g (per 100g) ✔

> ➢ Sodium content: 80mg (per 100g), 3% daily value based on a 2,000 calorie diet ✔
> ➢ Sugar content: 0g (per 100g) ✔

Allowed on the DASH diet. Ostrich is a meat option that is low in sodium and saturated fat.

Oyster:

> ➢ Saturated fat content: 3.2g (per 100g) 💀
> ➢ Sodium content: 417mg (per 100g), 17% daily value based on a 2,000 calorie diet 💀
> ➢ Sugar content: 0g (per 100g) ✔

Oysters are high in saturated fat and sodium. Try to limit or avoid on the DASH diet.

Papaya:

> ➢ Saturated fat content: 0.04g (per 100g) ✔
> ➢ Sodium content: 3mg (per 100g), less than 1% daily value based on a 2,000 calorie diet ✔
> ➢ Sugar content: 5.9g (per 100g) 💀

Papayas are high in lycopene and Vitamin C, which may help prevent heart disease. Include in moderation as part of a healthy diet.

Parsley:

> ➢ Saturated fat content: 0.1g (per 100g) ✔

➢ Sodium content: 56mg (per 100g), 2% daily value based on a 2,000 calorie diet ✔
➢ Sugar content: 0.9g (per 100g) ✔

Allowed on the DASH diet. Parsley is full of health boosting vitamins such as vitamin A, C, and K (source: *Real Simple*).

Parsnip:

➢ Saturated fat content: 0.1g (per 100g) ✔
➢ Sodium content: 10mg (per 100g), less than 1% daily value based on a 2,000 calorie diet ✔
➢ Sugar content: 4.8g (per 100g) ✔

Allowed on the DASH diet. Parsnips are rich in fiber and antioxidants (source: *BBC Good Food*).

Passionfruit:

➢ Saturated fat content: 0.1g (per 100g) ✔
➢ Sodium content: 28mg (per 100g), 1% daily value based on a 2,000 calorie diet ✔
➢ Sugar content: 11g (per 100g) ☠

Passionfruit is high in sugar. Try to limit or avoid on the DASH diet.

Pasta:

➢ Saturated fat content: 0.2g (per 100g) ✔

- ➢ Sodium content: 6mg (per 100g), less than 1% daily value based on a 2,000 calorie diet ✔
- ➢ Sugar content: 0.6g (per 100g) ✔

Allowed on the DASH diet. Choose wholegrain options when eating pasta.

Peach:

- ➢ Saturated fat content: 0.01g (per 100g) ✔
- ➢ Sodium content: 0mg (per 100g), less than 1% daily value based on a 2,000 calorie diet ✔
- ➢ Sugar content: 8.4g (per 100g) ☹

Some studies have shown that peaches contain compounds that may reduce the risk of heart disease (source: *Healthline*). Eat in moderation.

Peanuts:

- ➢ Saturated fat content: 7g (per 100g) ☹
- ➢ Sodium content: 18mg (per 100g) less than 1% daily value based on a 2,000 calorie diet ✔
- ➢ Sugar content: 4g (per 100g) ✔

Although nuts such as peanuts don't contain much sodium naturally, they're often sold covered in salt. Make sure to choose no-sodium or low sodium when purchasing them. In reality, it'll probably say 'unsalted' on the packet.

Pear:

➢ Saturated fat content: 0g (per 100g) ✔
➢ Sodium content: 1mg (per 100g), less than 1% daily value based on a 2,000 calorie diet ✔
➢ Sugar content: 10g (per 100g) 😧

Pears are high in sugar but rich in flavonoids that promote heart health and low blood pressure (source: *BBC Good Food*). Eat in moderation.

Peas (green):

➢ Saturated fat content: 0.1g (per 100g) ✔
➢ Sodium content: 5 mg (per 100g), less than 1% daily value based on a 2,000 calorie diet ✔
➢ Sugar content: 6g (per 100g) 😧

Peas contain omega-3 and omega-6 fatty acids that reduce oxidation and inflammation in the body (source: *WebMD*).

Pea Shoots (or pea sprouts):

➢ Saturated fat content: 0g ✔
➢ Sodium content: 0mg ✔
➢ Sugar content: 3g (per 70g) ✔

Allowed on the DASH diet. They're also a great source of fiber, vitamins A, C, and K and potassium (source: *Science Direct*).

Peppermint tea:

➢ Saturated fat content: 0g (per 100g) ✔
➢ Sodium content: 0mg (per 100g), 0% daily value based on a 2,000 calorie diet ✔
➢ Sugar content: 0g (per 100g) ✔

Allowed on the DASH diet. Choose teas such as peppermint tea as a healthier alternative to sugary drinks.

Pickled food:

➢ Saturated fat content: 0.082g (per 100g) ✔
➢ Sodium content: 1,061mg (per 100g) 😵
➢ Sugar content: 2.74g (per 100g) ✔

The above nutritional values are based on pickled vegetables from Fat Secret API's platform. Pickled foods are thought to be very high in sodium due to the brining process. Go for low-sodium options and eat in moderation.

Pineapple:

➢ Saturated fat content: 0g (per 100g) ✔
➢ Sodium content: 1mg (per 100g), less than 1% daily value based on a 2,000 calorie diet ✔
➢ Sugar content: 10g (per 100g) 😵

If you're buying canned fruits like pineapple, make sure you buy them canned in their own juice and not syrup to avoid extra sugar.

Pineapple is high in sugar, but can be consumed on occasion in the DASH diet.

Pistachio:

➢ Saturated fat content: 6g (per 100g) 😕
➢ Sodium content: 1mg (per 100g), less than 1% daily value based on a 2,000 calorie diet ✔
➢ Sugar content: 8g (per 100g) 😕

Pistachios are a heart healthy nut option. Eat in moderation as they're high in saturated fat and sugar.

Plum:

➢ Saturated fat content: 0g (per 100g) ✔
➢ Sodium content: 0mg (per 100g), less than 1% daily value based on a 2,000 calorie diet ✔
➢ Sugar content: 10g (per 100g) 😕

The potassium in plums are good for lowering blood pressure (source: *WebMD*). Include in moderation as a healthy part of the DASH diet.

Pomegranate:

➢ Saturated fat content: 0.1g (per 100g) ✔
➢ Sodium content: 3mg (per 100g), less 1% daily value based on a 2,000 calorie diet ✔
➢ Sugar content: 14g (per 100g) 😕

Pomegranate is high in sugar. Try to eat in moderation on the DASH diet.

Poppy seeds:

➢ Saturated fat content: 4.5 g (per 100g) 💀
➢ Sodium content: 26mg (per 100g), 1% daily value based on a 2,000 calorie diet ✔
➢ Sugar content: 3g (per 100g) ✔

Poppy seeds are high in saturated fat. Try to limit or avoid on the DASH diet.

Pork:

➢ Saturated fat content: 5g (per 100g) 💀
➢ Sodium content: 62mg (per 100g), 2% daily value based on a 2,000 calorie diet ✔
➢ Sugar content: 0g (per 100g) ✔

Pork is high in saturated fat. Try to choose leaner proteins like poultry on the DASH diet to limit fat intake.

Potato:

➢ Saturated fat content: 0.5g (per 100g) ✔
➢ Sodium content: 254mg (per 100g), 11% daily value based on a 2,000 calorie diet ✔
➢ Sugar content: 0.8g (per 100g) ✔

Potatoes are high in potassium, making them a good inclusion on the DASH diet (*CBS News)*. Eat in moderation to limit sodium intake.

Poultry meat:

➢ Saturated fat content: 7g (per 100g) 💀
➢ Sodium content: 40mg (per 100g), 1% daily value based on a 2,000 calorie diet ✔
➢ Sugar content: 0g (per 100g) ✔

Choose lean poultry meats like turkey and chicken on the DASH diet.

Prawn:

➢ Saturated fat content: 0.1g (per 100g) ✔
➢ Sodium content: 111mg (per 100g) 4% daily value based on a 2,000 calorie diet ✔
➢ Sugar content: 0g (per 100g) ✔

Allowed on the DASH diet. Prawns can be a great source of protein.

Processed cheese:

➢ Saturated fat content: 6g (per 100g) 💀
➢ Sodium content: 1,705mg (per 100g), 71% daily value based on a 2,000 calorie diet 💀
➢ Sugar content: 8g (per 100g) 💀

Try to limit or avoid intake of processed cheese on the DASH diet.

Prune:

➢ Saturated fat content: 0.1g (per 100g) ✔
➢ Sodium content: 2 mg (per 100g) less than 1% daily value based on a 2,000 calorie diet ✔
➢ Sugar content: 38g (per 100g) 💀

Prunes are high in sugar. Try to limit or avoid on the DASH diet.

Pulses:

➢ Saturated fat content: 0.1g (per 100g) ✔
➢ Sodium content: 5 mg (per 100g) less than 1% daily value based on a 2,000 calorie diet ✔
➢ Sugar content: 6g (per 100g) 💀

Pulses are high in sugar, so try to eat in moderation on the DASH diet.

Pumpkin seed oil:

➢ Saturated fat content: 10.1g (per 100g) 💀
➢ Sodium content: 0mg (per 100g) ✔
➢ Sugar content: 0mg (per 100g) ✔

(source: *Nutritionix*)

High in polyunsaturated fat, specifically omega-3s and omega-6 fatty acids. These are thought to be good fatty acids that raise good cholesterol and prevent heart disease (source: *Very Well Fit*).

Studies on post menopausal women have found a 2g dose of pumpkin seed oil per day for 12 weeks can decrease blood pressure (source: *https://clinicaltrials.gov/ct2/show/NCT02727036*)

Pumpkin seeds:

➢ Saturated fat content: 3.7g (per 100g) ✔
➢ Sodium content: 18mg (per 100g), less than 1% daily value based on a 2,000 calorie diet ✔
➢ Sugar content: 0g (per 100g) ✔

Allowed on the DASH diet. Pumpkin seeds are a healthy source of unsaturated fat (source: *BBC Good Food*).

Pumpkin:

➢ Saturated fat content: 0.1g (per 100g) ✔
➢ Sodium content: 1 mg (per 100g), less than 1% daily value based on a 2,000 calorie diet ✔
➢ Sugar content: 2.8g (per 100g) ✔

Allowed on the DASH diet. Pumpkin contains vitamin A and vitamin C, both vital for good health (source: *BBC Good Food*).

Quinoa:

➢ Saturated fat content: 0g (per 100g) ✔
➢ Sodium content: 5 mg (per 100g) less than 1% daily value based on a 2,000 calorie diet ✔
➢ Sugar content: 0.9g (per 100g) ✔

Allowed on the DASH diet. Add quinoa into your diet for a dose of healthy whole grains.

Rabbit:

➤ Saturated fat content: 2.5g (per 100g) 😲
➤ Sodium content: 199mg (per 100g) 9% daily value based on a 2,000 calorie diet ✔
➤ Sugar content: 0g (per 100g) ✔

Rabbit is high in saturated fat, so it may not be the best protein choice for the DASH diet.

Raclette cheese:

➤ Saturated fat content: 17.9g (per 100g) 😲
➤ Sodium content: 551mg (per 100g), 24% daily value based on a 2,000 calorie diet 😲
➤ Sugar content: 0.5g (per 100g) ✔

High in saturated fat and sodium. Avoid on the DASH diet.

Radish:

➤ Saturated fat content: 0g (per 100g) ✔
➤ Sodium content: 39mg (per 100g) 1% daily value based on a 2,000 calorie diet ✔
➤ Sugar content: 1.9g (per 100g) ✔

Allowed on the DASH diet. Radishes are ripe with antioxidants that can help protect and promote heart health (source: *Real Simple*).

Raisins:

➢ Saturated fat content: 0.1g (per 100g) ✔
➢ Sodium content: 11 mg (per 100g) less than 1% daily value based on a 2,000 calorie diet ✔
➢ Sugar content: 59g (per 100g) ☠

Raisins are high in sugar. Try to limit or avoid on the DASH diet.

Rapeseed oil (called canola oil in US):

➢ Saturated fat content: 8g (per 100g) ☠
➢ Sodium content: 0 mg (per 100g) 0% daily value based on a 2,000 calorie diet ✔
➢ Sugar content: 0g (per 100g) ✔

Rapeseed oil, also known as canola oil, is most often used as a cooking oil. Use in moderation due to the high saturated fat content.

Raspberry:

➢ Saturated fat content: 0g (per 100g) ✔
➢ Sodium content: 1g (per 100g), less than 1% daily value based on a 2,000 calorie diet ✔
➢ Sugar content: 4.4g (per 100g) ✔

Allowed on the DASH diet. Raspberries are a great source of vitamin C—just one cup provides more than 50% of the daily vitamin C target!

Raw milk:

➢ Saturated fat content: 3.7g (per 100g) 😲
➢ Sodium content: 40mg (per 100g) ✔
➢ Sugar content: Unknown

(source: *Slism*)

Milk that is unpasteurised. Note that all store bought milk is pasteurised. Raw milk is thought to be high in calcium content and fat. Go for skimmed or low-fat milk.

Red cabbage:

➢ Saturated fat content: 0g (per 100g) ✔
➢ Sodium content: 27 mg (per 100g) 1% daily value based on a 2,000 calorie diet ✔
➢ Sugar content: 3.8g (per 100g) ✔

Allowed on the DASH diet. Red cabbage is rich in antioxidants like anthocyanin that promote heart health (source: *BBC Good Food*).

Red wine vinegar:

➢ Saturated fat content: 0g (per 100g) ✔
➢ Sodium content: 8mg (per 100g), 1% daily value based on a 2,000 calorie diet ✔
➢ Sugar content: 0g (per 100g) ✔

(source: *Eat This Much*)

Allowed on the DASH diet. Red wine vinegar contains powerful antioxidants that promote heart health (source: *Healthline*).

Redcurrants:

➢ Saturated fat content: 0.2 g (per 100g) ✓
➢ Sodium content: 1 mg (per 100g) less than 1% daily value based on a 2,000 calorie diet ✓
➢ Sugar content: 7.4g (per 100g) ☠

Redcurrants are high in sugar. Try to avoid on the DASH diet.

Rhubarb:

➢ Saturated fat content: 0.1g (per 100g) ✓
➢ Sodium content: 4 mg (per 100g) less than 1% daily value based on a 2,000 calorie diet ✓
➢ Sugar content: 1.1g (per 100g) ✓

Allowed on the DASH diet. The high fiber content in rhubarb may be beneficial for heart health (source: *Verywell Fit*).

Rice:

➢ Saturated fat content: 0.1g (per 100g) ✓
➢ Sodium content: 1 mg (per 100g) less than 1% daily value based on a 2,000 calorie diet ✓
➢ Sugar content: 0.1g (per 100g) ✓

Allowed on the DASH diet. The DASH diet recommends several servings of whole grains per day.

Rice cakes:

➢ Saturated fat content: 0.57g (per 100g) ✔
➢ Sodium content: 326mg (per 100g) 💀
➢ Sugar content: 0.88g (per 100g) ✔

The above nutritional values are based on puffed rice cakes from Fat Secret API's platform. Rice cakes are thought to be high in sodium content. The amount of sodium varies by brand. Go for unsalted rice cakes.

Rice milk:

➢ Saturated fat content: 0g (per 100g) ✔
➢ Sodium content: 39 mg (per 100g), 1% daily value based on a 2,000 calorie diet ✔
➢ Sugar content: 5g (per 100g) 💀

Rice milk contains all the healthy nutrients that rice does. However, it lacks some of the protein that other milk choices like cow and soy provide (source: *Healthline*).

Rice noodles:

➢ Saturated fat content: 0g (per 100g) ✔
➢ Sodium content: 19 mg (per 100g), less than 1% daily value based on a 2,000 calorie diet ✔
➢ Sugar content: 0g (per 100g) ✔

Allowed on the DASH diet. Rice noodles can be a great source of complex carbohydrates, especially for those who are gluten-free (source: *Verywell Fit*).

Ricotta cheese:

➢ Saturated fat content: 8g (per 100g) 💀
➢ Sodium content: 84 mg (per 100g) 3% daily value based on a 2,000 calorie diet ✔
➢ Sugar content: 0.3g (per 100g) ✔

Ricotta cheese is high in saturated fat. Try to limit or avoid on the DASH diet.

Rooibos tea:

➢ Saturated fat content: 0g (per 100g) ✔
➢ Sodium content: 0g (per 100g), 0% daily value based on a 2,000 calorie diet ✔
➢ Sugar content: 0g (per 100g) ✔

(source: WebMD)

Allowed on DASH diet. A study suggested that rooibos tea may act as a natural blood pressure reducer (source: *WebMD*).

Roquefort cheese:

➢ Saturated fat content: 19.3g (per 100g) 💀
➢ Sodium content: 1809mg (per 100g) 79% daily value based on a 2,000 calorie diet 💀
➢ Sugar content: 0g (per 100g) ✔

High in saturated fat and sodium. Avoid on the DASH diet.

Rosemary:

➢ Saturated fat content: 2.8g (per 100g) ☹
➢ Sodium content: 26mg (per 100g) 1% daily value based on a 2,000 calorie diet ✓
➢ Sugar content: 0g (per 100g) ✓

Allowed on the DASH diet. Rosemary is rich in antioxidants that may help improve blood circulation (source: *Flushing Hospital*).

Rum:

➢ Saturated fat content: 0g (per 100g) ✓
➢ Sodium content: 1 mg (per 100g), less than 1% daily value based on a 2,000 calorie diet ✓
➢ Sugar content: 0g (per 100g) ✓

Limit alcoholic beverages when on the DASH diet.

Rye:

➢ Saturated fat content: 0.6g (per 100g) ✓
➢ Sodium content: 603 mg (per 100g) 25% daily value based on a 2,000 calorie diet ✓
➢ Sugar content: 3.9 g (per 100g) ✓

Rye is a wholegrain that is a great source of fiber. Rye bread is a nutritious choice for a daily serving of grains.

Sage:

➢ Saturated fat content: 7.03g (per 100g) 💀
➢ Sodium content: 11mg (per 100g), less than 1% daily value based on a 2,000 calorie diet ✔
➢ Sugar content: 1.7g (per 100g) ✔

Sage is an herb loaded with antioxidants. Use it to spruce up dishes with some added flavor.

Salami:

➢ Saturated fat content: 9 g (per 100g) 💀
➢ Sodium content: 1,740 mg (per 100g) 72% daily value based on a 2,000 calorie diet 💀
➢ Sugar content: 1g (per 100g) ✔

High in saturated fat and sodium. Try to limit or avoid on the DASH diet.

Salmon:

➢ Saturated fat content: 3.1g (per 100g) 💀
➢ Sodium content: 59 mg (per 100g) 2% daily value based on a 2,000 calorie diet ✔
➢ Sugar content: 0g (per 100g) ✔

Salmon is a great source of omega-3 fatty acids and potassium, both of which can help maintain blood pressure and contribute to heart health (source: *Safe Beat*).

Sauerkraut:

- ➤ Saturated fat content: 0g (per 100g) ✔
- ➤ Sodium content: 661 mg (per 100g), 27% daily value based on a 2,000 calorie diet ☺
- ➤ Sugar content: 1.8g (per 100g) ✔

Sauerkraut is high in sodium, but it is also full of healthy vitamins and minerals. Enjoy in moderation.

Sausages of all kinds:

- ➤ Saturated fat content: 11g (per 100g) ☺
- ➤ Sodium content: 731mg (per 100g) 30% daily value based on a 2,000 calorie diet ☺
- ➤ Sugar content: N/A

Avoid. Sausage is a processed meat high in saturated fat and sodium content. If you must eat meat, go for lean and low-fat meat.

Savoy cabbage:

- ➤ Saturated fat content: 0g (per 100g) ✔
- ➤ Sodium content: 28 mg (per 100g) 1% daily value based on a 2,000 calorie diet ✔
- ➤ Sugar content: 2.3g (per 100g) ✔

Cabbage is rich in vitamin B6 and folate, which are essential nutrients. Include cabbage in your diet to reach the 4-5 servings of vegetables a day.

Schnapps:

- ➢ Saturated fat content: 0g (per 100g) ✔
- ➢ Sodium content: 3mg (per 100g) ✔
- ➢ Sugar content: 4g (per 100g) ✔

The above nutritional values are based on Peach Schnapps from Calorie Counter's website. The sugar content varies depending on the flavour. Schnapps are thought to be high in calories. As Schnapps are a type of alcohol, watch consumption.

Seafood:

- ➢ Saturated fat content: 1.9g (per 100g) ✔
- ➢ Sodium content: 117mg (per 100g), 4% daily value based on a 2,000 calorie diet ✔
- ➢ Sugar content: N/A

The above nutritional values are based on roe from the USDA database. Check individual seafoods for specific nutritional values.

Seaweed:

- ➢ Saturated fat content: 0.1g (per 100g) ✔
- ➢ Sodium content: 102 mg (per 100g) 4% daily value based on a 2,000 calorie diet ✔
- ➢ Sugar content: 3g (per 100g) ✔

Seaweed is a great source of dietary iodine. Eat dried seaweed as a healthy snack or add fresh seaweed to cooked dishes.

Sesame:

➢ Saturated fat content: 7g (per 100g) ☠
➢ Sodium content: 11 mg (per 100g) less than 1% daily value based on a 2,000 calorie diet ✔
➢ Sugar content: 0.3g (per 100g) ✔

Sesame seeds are a rich source of protein and calcium. Consume in moderation as part of a healthy diet (source: *WebMD*).

Sheep's milk, sheep milk:

➢ Saturated fat content: 4.6g (per 100g) ☠
➢ Sodium content: 44 mg (per 100g) less than 1% daily value based on a 2,000 calorie diet ✔
➢ Sugar content: 0g (per 100g) ✔

Sheep's milk is an alternative to cow milk that is full of nutrients and protein. It is commonly used in some types of cheeses such as feta cheese. Consume in moderation due to the high fat content.

Shellfish:

See *bivalves*.

Shrimp:

➢ Saturated fat content: 0.1g (per 100g) ✔
➢ Sodium content: 111 mg (per 100g), 4% daily value based on a 2,000 calorie diet ✔
➢ Sugar content: 0g (per 100g) ✔

Also referred to as prawns. Shrimp is a great source of protein in a healthy diet.

Smoked fish:

➢ Saturated fat content: 0.9g (per 100g) ✔
➢ Sodium content: 780mg (per 100g), 34% daily value based on a 2,000 calorie diet ☠
➢ Sugar content: 0g (per 100g) ✔

High in sodium. Avoid all things smoked as salt is used in the smoking process.

Smoked meat:

➢ Saturated fat content: 0.9g (per 100g)
➢ Sodium content: 908.4mg (per 100g), 38% daily value based on a 2,000 calorie diet
➢ Sugar content: 0g (per 100g)

The above nutritional values are based on smoked ham from Nutritionix. Smoked meat includes sausages, bacon and ham to name a few. Avoid all things smoked as salt is used in the smoking process.

The National Cancer Institute notes a link between prostate, colon, rectal and pancreatic cancer and an increased intake of smoked meats.

Snow peas – see "green peas"

➢ Saturated fat content: 0.1g (per 100g) ✔
➢ Sodium content: 5 mg (per 100g) less than 1% daily value based on a 2,000 calorie diet ✔
➢ Sugar content: 6g (per 100g) 😵

Peas are rich in fiber and iron. They also contain heart healthy nutrients like potassium and calcium (source: *BBC Good Food*). Eat 4-5 servings of vegetables a day.

Soft cheese:

Brie

➢ Saturated fat content: 17g (per 100g) 😵
➢ Sodium content: 629mg (per 100g), 26% daily value based on a 2,000 calorie diet 😵
➢ Sugar content: 0.5g (per 100g) ✔

Camembert

➢ Saturated fat content: 15g (per 100g) 😵
➢ Sodium content: 842mg (per 100g), 35% daily value based on a 2,000 calorie diet 😵
➢ Sugar content: 0.5g (per 100g) ✔

Depends on the type of soft cheese. See the nutritional values for feta, cream cheese, roquefort and ricotta in this food list. Avoid brie and camembert as these are high in saturated fat and sodium content.

If you want cheese, Cleveland Clinic recommends going for naturally low-sodium cheese such as Swiss, goat, brick ricotta and fresh mozzarella.

Sour cream:

➤ Saturated fat content: 12g (per 100g) ☹
➤ Sodium content: 80 mg (per 100g), 3% daily value based on a 2,000 calorie diet ✓
➤ Sugar content: 2.9g (per 100g) ✓

Sour cream is high in saturated fat, so try to limit or avoid on the DASH diet.

Soy (soy beans, soy flour):

➤ Saturated fat content: 0.4g (per 100g) ✓
➤ Sodium content: 1,005 mg (per 100g), 41% daily value based on a 2,000 calorie diet ☹
➤ Sugar content: 0g (per 100g) ✓

Soy is a protein rich food that can often replace animal protein products in a diet. However, it can be high in sodium, so try to limit or avoid on the DASH diet.

Soy sauce:

➤ Saturated fat content: 0.1g (per 100g) ✓
➤ Sodium content: 5,493 mg (per 100g), 228% daily value based on a 2,000 calorie diet ☹
➤ Sugar content: 0.4g (per 100g) ✓

Soy sauce is generally high in sodium. Try to limit or avoid on the DASH diet.

Sparkling wine:

➢ Saturated fat content: 0g (per 100g) ✔
➢ Sodium content: 5mg (per 100g), less than 1% daily value based on a 2,000 calorie diet ✔
➢ Sugar content: 0.79g (per 100g) ✔

Drink alcohol sparingly on the DASH diet. You don't have to eliminate alcohol completely although it's good to limit consumption.

Spelt:

➢ Saturated fat content: 0.4g (per 100g) ✔
➢ Sodium content: 8 mg (per 100g), less than 1% daily value based on a 2,000 calorie diet ✔
➢ Sugar content: 7g (per 100g) ☻

Spelt is a type of grain similar to wheat. Include as one of your whole grain servings of the day.

Spinach:

➢ Saturated fat content: 0.06g (per 100g) ✔
➢ Sodium content: 79 mg (per 100g), 3% daily value based on a 2,000 calorie diet ✔
➢ Sugar content: 0.4g (per 100g) ✔

Spinach is an excellent vegetable to include on the DASH diet, containing vitamin K, potassium, and loads of antioxidants (source: *BBC Good Food*). Eat 4-5 servings of vegetables a day.

Spirits:

- ➢ Saturated fat content: 0g ✓
- ➢ Sodium content: 1mg, less than 1% daily value based on a 2,000 calorie diet ✓
- ➢ Sugar content: 0g ✓

Spirits include brandy, gin, tequila, whiskey, vodka and flavoured liquors (source: *The Spruce Eats*). Drink alcohol sparingly on the DASH diet. You don't have to eliminate alcohol completely although it's good to limit consumption.

Squashes:

Butternut squash

- ➢ Saturated fat content: 0g (per 100g) ✓
- ➢ Sodium content: 4mg (per 100g), less than 1% daily value based on a 2,000 calorie diet ✓
- ➢ Sugar content: 2.2g (per 100g) ✓

Spaghetti squash

- ➢ Saturated fat content: 0.1g (per 100g) ✓
- ➢ Sodium content: 17mg (per 100g), less than 1% daily value based on a 2,000 calorie diet ✓
- ➢ Sugar content: 2.8g (per 100g) ✓

Summer squash

➢ Saturated fat content: 0g (per 100g) ✔
➢ Sodium content: 2mg (per 100g), less than 1% daily value based on a 2,000 calorie diet ✔
➢ Sugar content: 2.2g (per 100g) ✔

Allowed on the DASH diet. I've listed a few above as examples. Try spaghetti squash instead of pasta to reduce the calories.

Stevia:

➢ Saturated fat content: 0g (per 100g) ✔
➢ Sodium content: 0g (per 100g), less than 1% daily value based on a 2,000 calorie diet ✔
➢ Sugar content: 0g (per 100g) ✔

Stevia is often used as a sugar substitute. Use it in coffee, tea, or baking instead of traditional sugar to cut back on sugar consumption.

Stinging nettle:

➢ Saturated fat content: 0g (per 100g) ✔
➢ Sodium content: 4 mg (per 100g) less than 1% daily value based on a 2,000 calorie diet ✔
➢ Sugar content: 0.3g (per 100g) ✔

Be sure to research the proper way to prepare stinging nettles before eating them, as they need to be cooked in order to become edible. But after that, stinging nettles are a healthy choice, chock full of vitamin A and vitamin C (source: *Eat Weeds*).

Strawberry:

➢ Saturated fat content: 0g (per 100g) ✔
➢ Sodium content: 1 mg (per 100g), less than 1% daily value based on a 2,000 calorie diet ✔
➢ Sugar content: 4.9g (per 100g) ✔

Strawberries are full of vitamin C and ripe with health benefits. Some studies suggest that strawberries may be helpful in a diet intended to reduce blood pressure.

Researchers conducted a large study with more than 34,000 people with hypertension.
They found that those with the highest intake of anthocyanins — mainly from blueberries and strawberries — had an 8 percent reduction in the risk of high blood pressure, compared to those with a low anthocyanin intake.

(source: *Medical News Today*)

Sugar:

➢ Saturated fat content: 0g (per 100g) ✔
➢ Sodium content: 1 mg (per 100g), less than 1% daily value based on a 2,000 calorie diet ✔
➢ Sugar content: 100g (per 100g) 💀

Try to limit sugar intake on the DASH diet.

Sunflower oil:

➢ Saturated fat content: 13g (per 100g) ☠
➢ Sodium content: 0mg (per 100g), less than 1% daily value based on a 2,000 calorie diet ✔
➢ Sugar content: 0g (per 100g) ✔

Sunflower oil is popular for cooking due to its high smoke point. However, it is high in saturated fats, so try to avoid on the DASH diet.

Sunflower seeds:

➢ Saturated fat content: 4.5g (per 100g) ☠
➢ Sodium content: 9 mg (per 100g), less than 1% daily value based on a 2,000 calorie diet ✔
➢ Sugar content: 2.6g (per 100g) ✔

Sunflower seeds are a great source of vitamin E, which protects the body from free radicals.

Sweetcorn:

➢ Saturated fat content: 0.2g (per 100g) ✔
➢ Sodium content: 15mg (per 100g), less than 1% daily value based on a 2,000 calorie diet ✔
➢ Sugar content: 3.2g (per 100g) ✔

Sweetcorn has a high fiber content, which may aid digestion and decrease risk of heart disease (source: *Birds Eye*).

Sweet potato:

➢ Saturated fat content: 0g (per 100g) ✔
➢ Sodium content: 55 mg (per 100g), less than 1% daily value based on a 2,000 calorie diet ✔
➢ Sugar content: 4.2g (per 100g) ✔

Also known as yams. Sweet potatoes are rich in potassium, making them helpful for lowering blood pressure (source: *Medical News Today*).

Tea, black:

➢ Saturated fat content: 0g (per 100g) ✔
➢ Sodium content: 3 mg (per 100g), less than 1% daily value based on a 2,000 calorie diet ✔
➢ Sugar content: 0g (per 100g) ✔

Black tea is full of antioxidants that may boost heart health. Drink it hot or iced, and refrain from adding any extra sugar to it.

Thyme:

➢ Saturated fat content: 0.5g (per 100g) ✔
➢ Sodium content: 9 mg (per 100g), less than 1% daily value based on a 2,000 calorie diet ✔
➢ Sugar content: 0g (per 100g) ✔

Thyme is a commonly used flavoring in meat, fish, and vegetable dishes. This herb has a multitude of healthy nutrients, such as potassium, vitamin A, and vitamin C (source: *WebMD*).

Tomato:

➢ Saturated fat content: 0g (per 100g) ✔
➢ Sodium content: 5mg (per 100g), less than 1% daily value based on a 2,000 calorie diet ✔
➢ Sugar content: 2.6g (per 100g) ✔

Tomatoes are high in lycopene, which may reduce the risk of heart disease. Tomatoes can be consumed in many different ways, from salads to sauces to sandwiches.

Trout:

➢ Saturated fat content: 1.4g (per 100g) ☹
➢ Sodium content: 51mg (per 100g), 2% daily value based on a 2,000 calorie diet ✔
➢ Sugar content: 0g (per 100g) ✔

Fish like trout are an excellent source of protein. Trout is low in mercury, making it a safe choice to include in a healthy diet (source: *SF Gate*).

Tuna:

➢ Saturated fat content: 0.4g (per 100g) ✔
➢ Sodium content: 47mg (per 100g), 1% daily value based on a 2,000 calorie diet ✔
➢ Sugar content: 0g (per 100g) ✔

Tuna is high in protein and B vitamins (source: *BBC Good Food*). Canned tuna can be eaten for convenience, or cook fresh tuna with vegetables for a delicious meal.

Turkey:

➢ Saturated fat content: 2.2g (per 100g) 😧
➢ Sodium content: 103mg (per 100g), 4% daily value based on a 2,000 calorie diet ✔
➢ Sugar content: 0g (per 100g) ✔

Turkey is a lean meat and a good choice for the DASH diet.

Turmeric:

➢ Saturated fat content: 3.1g (per 100g) 😧
➢ Sodium content: 38mg (per 100g), 1% daily value based on a 2,000 calorie diet ✔
➢ Sugar content: 3.2g (per 100g) ✔

Turmeric is a spice rich in health benefits. It contains natural anti-inflammatory compounds and antioxidants.

Turnip:

➢ Saturated fat content: 0g (per 100g) ✔
➢ Sodium content: 67mg (per 100g), 2% daily value based on a 2,000 calorie diet ✔
➢ Sugar content: 3.8g (per 100g) ✔

Turnips contain dietary nitrates that may help to reduce blood pressure, making them a fantastic food to include in the DASH diet (source: *Medical News Today*).

Vanilla:

➢ Saturated fat content: 0g (per 100g) ✔
➢ Sodium content: 9mg (per 100g), less than 1% daily value based on a 2,000 calorie diet ✔
➢ Sugar content: 13g (per 100g) 💀

Vanilla is often used as a flavoring in baked goods and desserts. It can be used as a substitute for sugar to add some sweetness to foods.

Venison:

➢ Saturated fat content: 1.3g (per 100g) 💀
➢ Sodium content: 54mg (per 100g), 2% daily value based on a 2,000 calorie diet ✔
➢ Sugar content: 0g (per 100g) ✔

Venison has more protein than any other red meat. It is also rich in iron (source: *The Guardian*). However, red meat should be limited or avoided on the DASH diet.

Vinegar: balsamic:

➢ Saturated fat content: 0g (per 100g) ✔
➢ Sodium content: 23mg (per 100g), less than 1% daily value based on a 2,000 calorie diet ✔
➢ Sugar content: 15g (per 100g) 💀

Some studies have suggested that balsamic vinegar can help to reduce cholesterol levels (source: *Healthline*).

Vinegar: distilled white vinegar:

➢ Saturated fat content: 0g (per 100g) ✔
➢ Sodium content: 2mg (per 100g), less than 1% daily value based on a 2,000 calorie diet ✔
➢ Sugar content: 0.04g (per 100g) ✔

Some studies suggest that consuming white vinegar may reduce blood sugar levels after a meal (source: *Healthline*).

Walnut:

➢ Saturated fat content: 6g (per 100g) ☹
➢ Sodium content: 2mg (per 100g) less than 1% daily value based on a 2,000 calorie diet ✔
➢ Sugar content: 2.6g (per 100g) ✔

Eatings nuts such as walnuts may help to lower blood pressure (source: *Healthline*). Choose walnuts as a healthy midday snack.

Watercress:

➢ Saturated fat content: 0g (per 100g) ✔
➢ Sodium content: 41mg (per 100g), 1% daily value based on a 2,000 calorie diet ✔
➢ Sugar content: 0.2g (per 100g) ✔

Watercress contains nitrates that can help to lower blood pressure (source: *Watercress*). Add it to your salad for a healthy boost.

Watermelon:

➢ Saturated fat content: 0g (per 100g) ✔
➢ Sodium content: 1mg (per 100g), less than 1% daily value based on a 2,000 calorie diet ✔
➢ Sugar content: 6g (per 100g) ☹

Watermelon is rich in three nutrients that can help reduce blood pressure—L-citrulline, lycopene, and potassium (source: *Eating Well*)

Wheat:

➢ Saturated fat content: 0.2g (per 100g) ✔
➢ Sodium content: 2mg (per 100g), less than 1% daily value based on a 2,000 calorie diet ✔
➢ Sugar content: 0.3g (per 100g) ✔

The DASH diet includes several servings of whole grains per day. Try to choose whole grains, which are rich in fiber and other nutrients (source: *Qardio*).

Wheat germ:

➢ Saturated fat content: 1.7g (per 100g) ☹
➢ Sodium content: 6mg (per 100g) less than 1% daily value based on a 2,000 calorie diet ✔
➢ Sugar content: 0g (per 100g) ✔

Wheat germ can be added to foods to increase nutritional value. High in fiber, wheat germ is packed with healthy nutrients. Try it on top of your oatmeal or yogurt, add it to a smoothie, or bake it into bread (source: *Bob's Red Mill*).

White button mushroom:

➢ Saturated fat content: 0.1g (per 100g) ✔
➢ Sodium content: 5mg (per 100g), less than 1% daily value based on a 2,000 calorie diet ✔
➢ Sugar content: 2g (per 100g) ✔

White button mushrooms are the most popular mushroom variety (source: *Mushroom Council*). Mushrooms can be prepared many ways and eaten with a wide variety of dishes, so they're easy to include in your diet. Try them sautéed with pasta or on top of pizza.

Wild rice:

➢ Saturated fat content: 0.2g (per 100g) ✔
➢ Sodium content: 7mg (per 100g), less than 1% daily value based on a 2,000 calorie diet ✔
➢ Sugar content: 2.5g (per 100g) ✔

Wild rice is actually not rice at all, but a species of grass that produces edible seeds that are similar to rice, hence the name! (source: *Healthline*). Wild rice is a powerful source of antioxidants and may be a heart healthy food to include in your diet.

Wine:

➢ Saturated fat content: 0g ✔
➢ Sodium content: 5mg (per 100g), less than 1% daily value based on a 2,000 calorie diet ✔
➢ Sugar content: 0.8g ✔

Drink alcohol sparingly on the DASH diet. You don't have to eliminate alcohol completely although it's good to limit consumption. A study found molecules in red wine may cause a drop in blood pressure (source: *British Heart Foundation*).

Many sources suggest red wine is high in antioxidants however, Dr. Robert Kloner, Chief Science Officer and Director of Cardiovascular Research at Huntington Medical Research Institutes argues the amount you need to drink for protective effects is debatable as this would mean drinking too much wine.

Yam:

➢ Saturated fat content: 0g (per 100g) ✔
➢ Sodium content: 9mg (per 100g), less than 1% daily value based on a 2,000 calorie diet ✔
➢ Sugar content: 0.5g (per 100g) ✔

Also known as sweet potatoes. Allowed on the DASH diet. Yams are a great source of fiber and vitamin C (source: *Fruits and Veggies*).

Yeast:

➢ Saturated fat content: 0.6g (per 100g) ✔
➢ Sodium content: 50mg (per 100g), 2% daily value based on a 2,000 calorie diet ✔
➢ Sugar content: 0g (per 100g) ✔

Allowed on the DASH diet. Yeast is often used in baking, particularly breads.

Yogurt/Yoghurt:

➢ Saturated fat content: 0.1g (per 100g) ✔
➢ Sodium content: 36mg (per 100g), 1% daily value based on a 2,000 calorie diet ✔
➢ Sugar content: 3.2g (per 100g) ✔

Low or nonfat yogurt can be a great choice to add to your diet. Enjoy it for breakfast or a snack, paired with fresh berries.

Zucchini:

➢ Saturated fat content: 0.1g (per 100g) ✔
➢ Sodium content: 8mg (per 100g), less than 1% daily value based on a 2,000 calorie diet ✔
➢ Sugar content: 2.5g (per 100g) ✔

Zucchini is rich in antioxidants and may promote heart health. Include zucchini as part of a well-rounded diet.

Printed in Great Britain
by Amazon

47169641R00076